Third Edition

3

CONSULTATION SKILLS FOR THE MRCGP

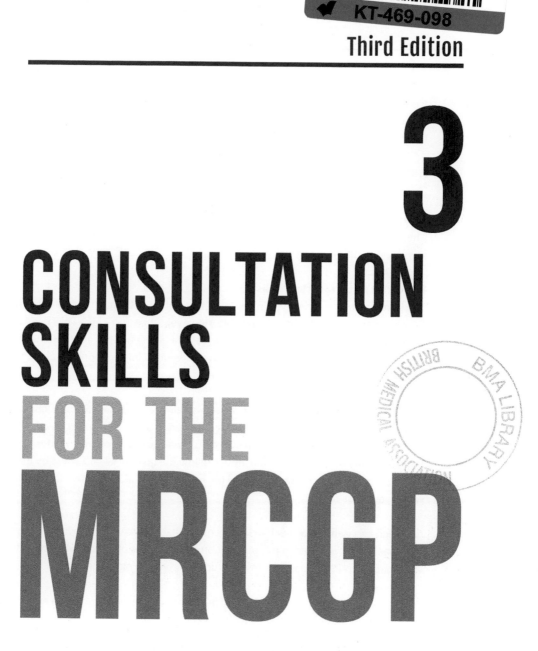

P. Naidoo MBChB, MRCGP, DRCOG, DFFP, Dip Occ, MSc
GP in Oxfordshire

Includes contributions from

C. Monkley MBBS, DRCOG, MSc (Sports Medicine), MRCGP, FFSEM (UK)
GP in the Defence Medical Services

Scion

© **Scion Publishing Limited, 2017**

First edition first published 2009; second edition published 2012

All rights reserved. No part of this book may be reproduced or transmitted, in any form or by any means, without permission.

A CIP catalogue record for this book is available from the British Library.

ISBN 9781911510031

Scion Publishing Limited

The Old Hayloft, Vantage Business Park, Bloxham Road, Banbury OX16 9UX, UK

www.scionpublishing.com

Important Note from the Publisher

The information contained within this book was obtained by Scion Publishing Ltd from sources believed by us to be reliable. However, while every effort has been made to ensure its accuracy, no responsibility for loss or injury whatsoever occasioned to any person acting or refraining from action as a result of information contained herein can be accepted by the authors or publishers.

Readers are reminded that medicine is a constantly evolving science and while the authors and publishers have ensured that all dosages, applications and practices are based on current indications, there may be specific practices which differ between communities. You should always follow the guidelines laid down by the manufacturers of specific products and the relevant authorities in the country in which you are practising.

Although every effort has been made to ensure that all owners of copyright material have been acknowledged in this publication, we would be pleased to acknowledge in subsequent reprints or editions any omissions brought to our attention.

Registered names, trademarks, etc. used in this book, even when not marked as such, are not to be considered unprotected by law.

Typeset by Phoenix Photosetting, Chatham, Kent, UK

Printed in the UK

Contents

Preface to the third edition

When this book was published in its first and second editions, as a companion guide to *Cases and Concepts for the new MRCGP* (2009), it included a DVD. The DVD featured thirteen GP consultations, and trainees were asked to mark the consultation according to a CSA marking schedule. I thought the DVD would be used for group work. I had observed that trainees were often reluctant to bring their own video consultations for group work and were understandably sensitive to feedback. I assumed that producing DVDs, featuring variable standards of consulting, would facilitate case marking and stimulate discussion on how performance could be improved. Unfortunately, several readers assumed that the DVD featured examples of excellent consulting, and mistook it for a 'how to' guide, which was not the intention at all. For this reason, I have omitted the DVD from this edition and replaced the thirteen Video cases with thirteen Teaching cases.

The thirteen Teaching cases are very detailed and follow a particular format.
- Information for the doctor: this would be the printout that the candidate is handed, to read through before the patient enters the consulting room.
- Information for the actor / patient: this provides the actor with sufficient information to convincingly become the patient.
- Suggested approach to the consultation: this highlights the data gathering, management and interpersonal skills this case requires. This is the 'model answer'.
- The case ends with the background knowledge required for this case, or the theory underpinning the consultation. In addition, I supply references and signpost to various sources of information. Guidelines change quickly, so I provide the most up-to-date guidance at the time of writing. This allows you to understand how I made my judgements and wrote my marking schedules.

Once candidates learn from the thirteen Teaching cases, they are presented with twenty complete Long cases, designed to aid them in CSA preparation. Each of the twenty cases features detailed analysis to demonstrate to candidates an ordered, step-wise approach to data gathering, clinical management and interpersonal skills. It is important to learn and practise these skills, but the trainee who tries to practise every potential examination case to get the 'answer right' is embarking on a long and exhausting journey. It may be a more efficient use of time to recognise a type of case and to have a methodical approach.

For example, some cases are written to be ethical dilemmas; others are cases where the patient presents with a request, i.e. the solution which they think is the answer to their clinical problem. If you recognise the type of case (for example, patient presents with a specific request), work out what you need to demonstrate (for example, thorough assessment of the underlying problem, a choice of options the patient may not have considered, arguments for and against the specific request). If you recognise the type of case and roll out your methodical approach, you do not have to practise every mock CSA case written around this permutation. Think of skilled learner drivers who have practised hill starts, urban and rural traffic – they do not try to drive down every possible road before the driving test. Success depends on recognising a hill start and deploying your pre-planned strategy, which you have practised on several previous occasions.

With this in mind, the book is useful to Specialist Trainees (ST) in general practice right from the start of their training.

- ST1s will find the thirteen Teaching cases most useful.
- ST2s, reading the analysis and discussion in the Long cases, will be prepared for COT discussions.
- ST3s preparing for the CSA could use the Teaching and Long cases for revision and the final section of the book, Practice cases, for group study. The Practice cases cover typical CSA cases, such as paediatric and telephone consultations, dealing with lists, breaking bad news, and home visits.

Best wishes with your examination preparation and good luck!

Dr P. Naidoo
January 2017

Acknowledgments

Thank you to my trainees: you have inspired and challenged.

The Defence Deanery: thank you for taking me into your fold. Your support and encouragement have meant a lot to me.

Julie Stokes: thank you for the lunchtime runs, an opportunity to shed calories and clear the cobwebs.

Finally, to my husband Anton – have faith, I'm sure the Boks will make a spectacular comeback.

Dedication

This book is dedicated to my mother who has enjoyed teaching for more than 40 years, a hard act to follow.

Abbreviations

A&E	Accident and Emergency department
AA	Alcoholics Anonymous
ACR	Albumin–creatinine ratio
ACS	Acute coronary syndrome
AF	Atrial fibrillation
AIDS	Acquired immune deficiency syndrome
ALT	Alanine transaminase
ARB	Angiotensin receptor blocker
AV	Atrioventricular
BCC	Basal cell carcinoma
BD	Twice a day
BG	Blood glucose
BMI	Body mass index
BP	Blood pressure
BPE	Benign prostatic enlargement
BPPV	Benign paroxysmal positional vertigo
bpm	Beats per minute
CBT	Cognitive behavioural therapy
CHC	Combined hormonal contraceptive
CKD	Chronic kidney disease
CLE	Continuous laryngoscopy exercise
CMH	Community Mental Health
CNS	Central nervous system
COC	Combined oral contraceptive
COPD	Chronic obstructive pulmonary disease
CRP	C-reactive protein
CSA	Clinical Skills Assessment
CTS	Carpal tunnel syndrome
CVS	Cardiovascular system
CXR	Chest X-ray
D&V	Diarrhoea and vomiting
DEXA	Dual-energy X-ray absorptiometry
DN	District Nurse
DoH	Department of Health
DSH	Deliberate self-harm
DVLA	Driver and Vehicle Licensing Agency
DVT	Deep vein thrombosis
ECG	Electrocardiogram
EIB	Exercise-induced bronchoconstriction
EILO	Exercise-induced laryngeal obstruction
ENT	Ear, nose and throat
ESR	Erythrocyte sedimentation rate
FBC	Full blood count
FH	Familial hypercholesterolaemia
GA	General anaesthetic
GFR	Glomerular filtration rate
GI	Gastrointestinal
GMC	General Medical Council
GORD	Gastro-oesophageal reflux disease
Hb	Haemoglobin
HBV	Hepatitis B virus
hCG	Human chorionic gonadotrophin
HDL	High-density lipoprotein
HIV	Human immunodeficiency virus
HMB	Heavy menstrual bleeding
HRT	Hormone replacement therapy
HS	Heart sounds
HV	Health visitor
IBD	Inflammatory bowel disease
IBS	Irritable bowel syndrome
ICSI	Intracytoplasmic sperm injection
IHD	Ischaemic heart disease
IM	Intramuscular
IUD	Intrauterine device (e.g. copper coil)
IUS	Intrauterine system (e.g. Mirena)
IV	Intravenous
IVF	*In vitro* fertilisation

LDL	Low-density lipoprotein	PR	*per rectum*
LFTs	Liver function tests	PRN	As required
LMP	Last menstrual period	PSA	Prostate-specific antigen
LUTI	Lower urinary tract infection	PT	Prothrombin time
LUTS	Lower urinary tract symptoms	PV	*per vagina*
MC&S	Microscopy, culture and sensitivities	QDS	Four times a day
		RCT	Randomised controlled trial
MCH	Mean cell haemoglobin	RS	Respiratory system
MCV	Mean corpuscular volume	SARS	Sudden acute respiratory syndrome
MDU	Medical Defence Union		
MI	Myocardial infarction	SGPT	Serum glutamic-pyruvic transaminase
MS	Multiple sclerosis		
MSU	Mid-stream urine	SHBG	Sex hormone binding globulin
MT	Metatarsal	SIGN	Scottish Intercollegiate Guidelines Network
MTP	Metatarsophalangeal		
NAD	No abnormality detected	SLE	Systemic lupus erythematosus
NAI	Non-accidental injury	SSRI	Selective serotonin reuptake inhibitor
NICE	National Institute for Health and Care Excellence		
		STD	Sexually transmitted disease
NSAID	Non-steroidal anti-inflammatory drug	STI	Sexually transmitted infection
		SVT	Supraventricular tachycardia
NVD	Normal vaginal delivery	TCA	Tricyclic antidepressant
OAB	Overactive bladder	TDS	Three times a day
OC	Obstetric cholestasis	TFTs	Thyroid function tests
OCD	Obsessive–compulsive disorder	TIA	Transient ischaemic attack
OD	Once a day	TOP	Termination of pregnancy
OPD	Outpatient department	TPO	Thyroid peroxidase
OTC	Over-the-counter	TSH	Thyroid-stimulating hormone
O/E	On examination	U&Es	Urea and electrolytes
ON	Ophthalmia neonatorum	UC	Ulcerative colitis
PAAP	Personal asthma action plan	UKMEC	UK Medical Eligibility Criteria
PCOS	Polycystic ovary syndrome	URTI	Upper respiratory tract infection
PE	Pulmonary embolism		
PF	Plantar fasciitis	USS	Ultrasound scan
POP	Progesterone-only contraceptive pill	UTI	Urinary tract infection
		VE	Vaginal examination
PPH	Post-partum haemorrhage	VT	Ventricular tachycardia
PPT	Post-partum thyroiditis	WBC	White blood count

Web links

There are many online references throughout this book signposting readers to up-to-date resources. Where these are long, we have created a 'tiny url' so that the relevant website can be accessed without having to key in a long web address.

Take, for example, a long weblink such as https://www.nice.org.uk/guidance/ng12/chapter/1-Recommendations-organised-by-site-of-cancer#lower-gastrointestinal-tract-cancers which appears in Long case 12.

This would appear in the text as:

tinyurl.com/CS3e-Lc12a (*takes you to* www.nice.org.uk/guidance/ng12/...)

Teaching case 1 – Child

Information for the doctor

Name	Kristina Hood	
Date of birth (Age)	21 months	
Social and Family History	Has a 3 year old sister	
Past medical history	2 months ago	Otitis media
	6 months ago	Croup
	8 months ago	Enlarged lymph node
	14 months ago	Chickenpox
	18 months ago	GORD
Past medication	Gaviscon	

Information for the mother

You are Gemma, the concerned mother of 21 month old Kristina, who has called the doctor to discuss Kristina's ongoing vomiting since her fall from a sofa 5 days ago. You were in the kitchen and the girls were in the living room. You think Kristina may have been standing on the sofa and was pushed off by her sister. She cried immediately and vomited 30 minutes later. You took her to the ED where she had a CT head scan. You were told the scan was clear. Since the head injury, Kristina vomits more often, she is irritable and clingy and her behaviour has changed.

You think that Kristina suffered a brain injury or has a recurrence of her reflux causing her vomiting. Your opening statement is *"I'm really worried about Kristina's vomiting. I thought she would be better by now."*

Information to reveal if asked

General information about Kristina, including occupation:
- You are a stay-at-home mum and Kristina has been healthy since her troublesome GORD in early infancy. Gaviscon caused constipation in the past.

Further details about Kristina's condition:
- If specifically asked about the vomiting, Kristina vomits once immediately after the evening meal at 5pm and in the night at 1am. She passes one semi-formed stool; the frequency is normal but the consistency has changed. She is eating and drinking well.
- If asked about her behaviour, she is a lot more irritable with her sister, clingy with mum and 'irritable'.

Your ideas about the illness, your treatment preferences, your coping skills and beliefs about healthcare:

- You think that Kristina may have reflux again. The ED doctors examined her thoroughly and checked for a temperature, rash and infection but all was well. In between clingy crying behaviour, Kristina is boisterous and happy.

Your concerns about the illness, treatments, prognosis and length of illness:

- You are worried that the CT scan may have missed a small problem and Kristina may have a brain problem. You don't want to wait too long in case it is getting worse.

Your expectations of the consultation and of treatment:

- You expect to be offered an appointment for Kristina to be examined.

Suggested approach to the telephone consultation

Targeted history taking:

- Take a detailed history of Kristina's symptoms:
  - two episodes of vomiting per day
  - altered behaviour: irritability and clinginess interspersed with normal behaviour.
- Explore mum's ideas about why she thinks this is reflux and if she expects a script for Gaviscon.
- Mum stated her concerns at the outset. Explore her fears about a missed brain injury.
- Explore her expectations – how does she want Kristina re-evaluated?
- Explore the possible causes of vomiting and changed behaviour in greater detail – take a good history to assess the likelihood of infection or neurological problems.
- Discuss a possible diagnosis of concussion.
- Offer options such as a GP review appointment or a 'watch and call back'.
- Address the mum's ideas that this could be reflux. Discuss the symptoms of concussion.
- Address the mum's concerns about a missed head injury. Discuss how a diagnosis of concussion is made.
- Address the mum's expectations of a review: offer a face-to-face check for signs of head injury, infection and behaviour/social interaction.
- Confirm mum's understanding of concussion – consider signposting to an online patient information leaflet.
- Arrange suitable follow-up.

Interpersonal skills:

This case tests the doctor's ability to explore a presenting problem more deeply, eliciting the absence of 'head injury red flags', resulting in the diagnosis of concussion. It also tests the doctor's ability to explain the diagnosis to a worried mum.

Good communication with the patient:
- Encourages mum to explore Kristina's symptoms through the skilful use of open questions: *"I'm really interested in the changed behaviour – give me examples of clinginess/irritability. What happens in between these bouts?"*
- Makes statements to explore understanding of the tentative diagnosis (concussion): *"Based on Kristina's history and the hospital's examination findings, this is most likely concussion. What is your understanding of concussion? Do you know anyone who has had concussion?"*
- Encourages reflection: *"Based on the information you have given me, this sounds like concussion. Do you want me to tell you where you can look up some information on concussion? How do you feel about this?"*
- Builds trust through reflective listening: *"It sounds like you, like any concerned parent, are scared of the possibility of brain damage. Shall we make an appointment to examine Kristina thoroughly? How does that sound?"*

Poor communication with the patient:
- Asks a series of closed questions without putting them in context for mum, which could increase her anxiety.
- Fails to discuss 'concussion'. Without this information, mum is not empowered to amend her concerns and expectations.
- Is prescriptive in their management: *"Just read the patient information leaflet and stop worrying."*

Background knowledge required for this case

A child presenting with 'red flag' features after a head injury warrants prolonged observation.

Red flag symptoms:

- Complaints of neck pain
- Increasing confusion or irritability
- Repeated vomiting
- Seizure or convulsion
- Weakness or tingling/burning in arms or legs
- Deteriorating conscious state
- Severe or increasing headache
- Unusual behaviour/change in behaviour
- Diplopia.

Children should be reviewed if symptoms persist for 7–10 days as well as prior to returning to any exercise and prior to returning to contact sport.

The recovery from concussion in children generally occurs over a longer time period than in adults. This is evident in time for symptom resolution, as well as neurocognitive recovery. On average, sports-concussed high school athletes take twice as long to recover (10–14 days) as college and professional athletes (3–7 days), and pre-adolescent children may take even longer to recover. These effects may have significant impact on the child's ability to return to school because of the concussive neurocognitive deficits such as slowed information processing, difficulty forming new memory and inability to concentrate.

Cognitive rest includes limiting any activity requiring concentration and attention which exacerbates symptoms, including television, video/electronic games, texting, computer work and reading. Participation in these activities ('cognitive overexertion') may increase concussion symptoms and prolong recovery.

NICE (2014) *Head Injury: assessment and early management guideline* (CG 176): www.nice.org.uk/guidance/cg176

Teaching case 2 – Adult man

Information for the doctor

Name	Suresh Pillai
Date of birth (Age)	45
Social and Family History	Married, two teenage children
Past medical history	1 year ago Knee pain
	1 year ago Shingles
	3 years ago Clavicle fracture
	12 years ago Urethral stricture

Information for the patient

You are Suresh Pillai, a 45-year-old security guard who has come to the doctor with a month-long history of left elbow pain (you are left-handed). The pain started after a 3-day team-building event where you and your colleagues did a 'boot camp'. This involved abseiling, cycling, low ropes, high ropes and camping.

You present to the doctor expecting to discuss medication because resting the elbow and ibuprofen did not work. You are working night shifts for the next month and then you are taking a long holiday to India to visit your family. Your opening statement is *"My elbow is sore but I'm too young for arthritis, doctor."*

Information to reveal if asked

General information about yourself, including occupation:
- You work as a security guard for a large security company, rotating buildings and shifts. Some shifts, especially night shifts, involve patrols to check that areas are properly locked and things are secured.
- You clay pigeon shoot with friends. Firing the rifle has become painful (7/10).

Further details about your condition:
- The left elbow pain started about a month ago after the team-building exercise.
- The pain is a dull ache (2/10) in the left upper arm in the morning, but 7/10 after a busy shift. It is really sore 6/10 when rubbed. It is worse (6/10) when you carry the shopping and check to see if a door is locked. Ibuprofen helps but the pain returns.
- You do not experience weakness or pins and needles.
- You have not injured the elbow, or shoulder or neck, in the past.
- Some relatives take medication for 'arthritis' but you have kept yourself reasonably fit. You cycle on a stationary bike at work three times per week and you walk a lot in your work.

Your ideas about the illness, your treatment preferences, your coping skills and beliefs about healthcare:

- You think that you hurt the elbow during the team-building exercise but you are worried about arthritis and would like to be examined.
- You think stronger tablets may help but you are not keen on taking daily tablets. If the doctor offers you patches, you are very interested in this.
- You spoke to a co-worker who said a brace could be helpful. Perhaps you could get a letter asking the company to pay for a brace.

Your concerns about the illness, treatments, prognosis, length of illness, effects on their work and role:

- You are worried about elbow arthritis and long-term damage.

Your expectations of the consultation and of treatment:

- You expect to get treatment that ties in with your shift patterns and imminent holiday.
- If the doctor thinks a brace would be helpful, you'd like a letter for a brace.

Information to reveal when examined

If the doctor asks to examine your elbow, you are tender in left epicondyle and forearm extensors, where the pain worsens with resisted L wrist extension.

You are not overweight.

See tinyurl.com/CS3e-Tc2a (*takes you to* www.sportsinjuryclinic.net/.../tennis-elbow-assessment)

Suggested approach to the consultation

Targeted history taking:

- What are Suresh's symptoms? Has he tried rest and anti-inflammatories? Did he experience any side-effects from the anti-inflammatories?
- What does he suspect is causing his left elbow pain? Has he heard of 'tennis elbow'? What does he understand about the natural history and treatment of tennis elbow?
- What are his concerns? Why is he worried about elbow arthritis? Is he worried about long-term treatment and how helpful tablets may be in 'curing' the problem?
- What treatment options would he prefer – relative rest and daily frictional massage with NSAID gel; oral NSAIDs; physiotherapy for exercises and assessment of a brace; referral to a colleague for a steroid injection; off-licence use of GTN patches daily for six weeks?

Targeted examination:

Elbow examination as per tinyurl.com/CS3e-Tc2a (*takes you to* www.
sportsinjuryclinic.net/.../tennis-elbow-assessment)

Clinical management:

- The doctor could address the patient's concerns about arthritis and simultaneously explore red flags, by asking about morning stiffness, swelling, multiple joint involvement and systemic symptoms. This set of questions could be signposted by saying, *"To rule out serious illness, such as arthritis, I need to ask you a few quick questions. Are your joints stiff in the morning; do you have pain in the..."*
- The doctor, based on the typical history and examination findings, confirms a working diagnosis of tennis elbow and explains the condition.
- The doctor explores Mr Pillai's idea that the pain was brought on by the team-building exercises by discussing how repetitive movements could aggravate the condition. Tennis elbow may take 6–12 months to get better.
- Negotiates a letter for the company. The letter could advise on avoiding tasks involving lifting, gripping, pronation and supination and advises taking regular breaks.
- The doctor could offer a referral to physiotherapy for the physiotherapist to assess whether a brace is needed and to choose the most suitable brace (NHS funded). Alternatively the wording of a letter for the company for a tennis elbow off-loading brace could be negotiated.
- Addresses his expectations for practical advice: discusses treatment options (www. aafp.org/afp/2007/0915/p843.html). Topical and oral NSAIDs are useful in the first month, after which it may be reasonable to switch to paracetamol with or without codeine. As Mr Pillai is not easily available for further medical appointments in the next two months, the off-licence use of GTN patches may be an attractive option for him. One RCT of 86 patients compared a nitroglycerin transdermal patch with a placebo patch. The nitroglycerin patch reduced elbow pain with activity at 2 weeks, and reduced epicondylar tenderness at 6 and 12 weeks. At 6 months, 81% of treated patients were asymptomatic during activities of daily living.
- Provides some information on the pros and cons of GTN patches and steroid injection, which, if expertise is available in Primary Care, may be useful for short-term relief of severe pain.
- Provides information on the natural history of tennis elbow and discusses follow-up.

Interpersonal skills:

This case tests the doctor's ability to inform a patient about a new diagnosis (tennis elbow) and devise a treatment plan (GTN patches or steroid + local anaesthetic injections) in keeping with his travel plans.

Good communication with the patient:

- Establishes rapport by listening attentively to Mr Pillai's opening statements and acknowledging his fears about having developed a long-term, 'incurable' illness ('arthritis').
- Displays empathy to his fixed travel plans and offers treatment compatible with his time scales.
- Encourages autonomy and opinions – provides him with treatment options, discussing their risks and benefits and facilitating the patient's choice.
- Good prescribing behaviour involves discussing how NSAIDs should be used in a chronic condition such as tennis elbow and discussing alternative analgesia.
- Good negotiation skills are required to deal with his request for a company letter for a 'brace'.

Background knowledge required for this case

Johnson GW *et al.* (2007) Treatment of lateral epicondylitis. *American Family Physician*, **76(6):** 843–8: www.aafp.org/afp/2007/0915/p843.html

Repetitive wrist dorsiflexion with supination and pronation causes overuse of the extensor tendons of the forearm and subsequent microtears, collagen degeneration, and angiofibroblastic proliferation. If untreated, lateral epicondylitis persists for an average of 6–24 months.

Topical NSAIDs may provide short-term (up to 3 weeks) pain relief.

Patients receiving corticosteroid injections showed greater perception of benefit at 4 weeks than patients receiving oral NSAIDs (such as naproxen 500 mg OD or BD), but this benefit did not persist in the longer term.

Local corticosteroid injection has short-term (2–6 weeks) benefits in pain reduction, global improvement, and grip strength.

Use of an inelastic, non-articular, proximal forearm strap may decrease pain and increase grip strength after 3 weeks. Bracing for up to 6 weeks also may improve the patient's ability to perform daily activities.

More data are needed before acupuncture or botulinum toxin type A injection can be recommended to treat lateral epicondylitis.

Treatment of lateral epicondylitis

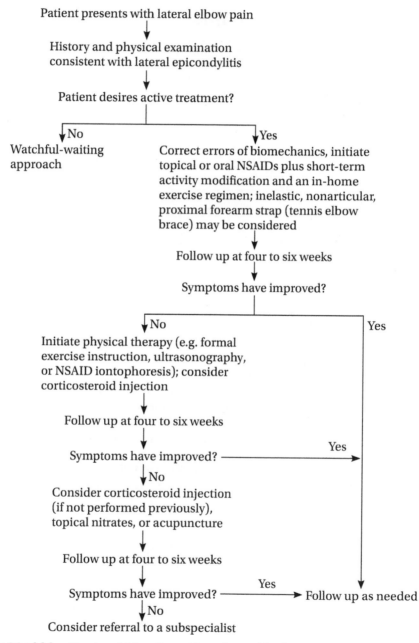

Patient presents with lateral elbow pain

History and physical examination
consistent with lateral epicondylitis

Patient desires active treatment?

No — Watchful-waiting approach

Yes — Correct errors of biomechanics, initiate topical or oral NSAIDs plus short-term activity modification and an in-home exercise regimen; inelastic, nonarticular, proximal forearm strap (tennis elbow brace) may be considered

Follow up at four to six weeks

Symptoms have improved?

No — Initiate physical therapy (e.g. formal exercise instruction, ultrasonography, or NSAID iontophoresis); consider corticosteroid injection

Yes

Follow up at four to six weeks

Symptoms have improved? — Yes

No — Consider corticosteroid injection (if not performed previously), topical nitrates, or acupuncture

Follow up at four to six weeks

Symptoms have improved? — Yes → Follow up as needed

No — Consider referral to a subspecialist

NOTE: *Watchful waiting is a viable option and may be considered at any step.*

Reproduced with permission from the American Academy of Family Physicians, from Johnson, G.W. *et al.* Treatment of lateral epicondylitis. *Am. Fam. Physician* (2007) **76(6):** 843–8.

Teaching case 3 – Teenage boy

Information for the doctor

Name	James Preston
Date of birth (Age)	15
Social and Family History	Lives with mum and stepdad. Has 2 younger half-siblings
Past medical history	1 year ago Injury from rugby 18 months ago Eczema 3 years ago Allergic rhinitis
Past medication	Dermol ointment, apply as emollient to dry skin

Information for the patient

You are James Preston, a 15 year old student, who has come to discuss the head injury you sustained during a school hockey game yesterday. You attend with your mum, who sits quietly in the room. At 11.45am yesterday, you, with a team member, were moving a hockey goal into position for a game, when someone threw the hockey ball into the air and aimed for the goal. The hockey ball hit you on the side of the face, just above your left ear. You fell to the ground with your eyes closed, in severe pain. You could hear your friend and teacher talking but the pain was so bad (8/10) that you couldn't focus on what they were saying. You remember being helped to the nurse's room where you rested for a while. While in her room, you remember looking down at your feet and they looked as if they were spinning. This only lasted a few seconds and you have not experienced any further episodes of dizziness. The pain gradually reduced to 4/10 with paracetamol and is now mild (3/10). You have a mild headache, pain in the R jaw, no clicking of the jaw; no problems chewing and no nausea.

You think that you may have hurt your jaw but your mum is worried about a head injury and whether you should play your game at the weekend (in 3 days). Your opening statement is *"I think I'm OK but just wanted to be checked out because mum is worrying."*

Information to reveal if asked

General information about yourself, including occupation:
- You are at school – no problems.
- You enjoy sport. You are not competitive at high levels, just for fun.

Further details about your condition:
- If specifically asked about the injury, you don't think you lost consciousness. You closed your eyes from the pain, but you were dimly aware of the conversation around you. Your teacher didn't think you had lost consciousness.

- If asked about the headache, most of the pain is just above your jaw near the scalp, but you do not have any bruising or cuts. You took paracetamol but your mum wouldn't give you ibuprofen in case you had an internal bleed. The pain is manageable; more of a dull ache.
- You are usually fit and healthy.

Your ideas about the illness, your treatment preferences, your coping skills and beliefs about healthcare:
- You think that you were lucky and had a minor sports injury.

Your concerns about the illness, treatments, prognosis and length of illness:
- Your mum is worried that you have a minor head injury. She looked it up on the internet and thinks the headache, dizziness and possible loss of consciousness should be taken seriously.

Your expectations of the consultation and of treatment:
- You expect to be advised about whether you can compete in Saturday's game.

Information to reveal if examined

You have slight tenderness on the face above the R temporomandibular joint.

On completing SCAT-2 (http://bjsm.bmj.com/content/43/Suppl_1/i85.full.pdf), you:
- are fully orientated
- get 3 answers incorrect on recall scoring 12/15
- score 5/5 for concentration
- score full marks on balance testing
- score full marks for coordination testing
- score 3/5 for delayed recall.

Suggested approach to the consultation

Targeted history taking:

- Take a detailed history of:
  - mechanism of injury
  - presence of symptoms, such as headache, nausea, balance problems, confusion, irritability, difficulties with concentrating or remembering, not feeling 'himself/right'.
- Explore James's ideas about this being 'minor'. What would make it a 'bad' injury?
- James stated his mum's concern about this being a minor head injury. Discuss what 'concussion' is and how you clinically intend to assess for it and stratify its severity.
- Explore his expectations – should he play competitive sport in 3 days?

Targeted examination:

- Check for skull or facial bone fracture or a local soft tissue injury.
- Perform an examination designed to tell you how well the brain is working:
    - is he orientated? (particularly in time)
    - can he remember? (ask him to recall a list of 5 words)
    - can he concentrate? (recite the months backwards)
    - can he balance (on both legs and on one leg) with eyes open and closed?
    - assess coordination using the finger to nose test
    - can he recall the original list of 5 words?

Clinical management:

- Discuss that based on history and examination, he has mild concussion. Advise 24 hours complete rest at home – no computing / homework / studying / sport.
- Discuss the need for observation for the first 24–48 hours. If he develops red flags (severe / worsening headache, confusion / drowsiness / unsteadiness / slurred speech), he needs to attend hospital at once.
- Discuss a graduated return to play, from rest until asymptomatic to light exercise (stationary bike) to sport-specific exercise to non-contact then contact drills, then contact training leading to competitive games.
- Address James's idea that he has a minor injury. Discuss 'minor concussion'.
- Address the patient's concerns about returning to competitive sport. *"I think we need to take this injury seriously. Most athletes do better when they have a graduated return to sport. What do you think about missing Saturday's game and getting back into things a bit more gently?"*
- Address the patient's expectations: give advice about a return to play and red flags.
- Confirm his understanding of concussion and its treatment options – consider a patient information leaflet.
- Arrange suitable follow-up, possibly with medical cover at the games so that he is cleared fit before he plays.

Interpersonal skills:

This is a relatively simple case of concussion. Once 'red flags' are actively excluded, the diagnosis is not difficult to make. The doctor's ability to reassure, particularly through the use of systematic examination, is tested. The concerns about safety to return to sport are addressed, using evidence-based guidelines.

Good communication with the patient:
- Encourages the patient to explore his symptoms through the skilful use of open questions: *"Tell me what happened after the ball struck your face. Besides the pain, what else were you aware of? When your eyes were closed, what could you hear?"*
- Signposts aspects of the examination and interprets the findings to the patient and his mum.

- Builds trust through reflective listening: *"It sounds like your mum is concerned about you returning to sport too soon, without giving your brain enough time to recover from this knock. What do you think could happen if you got a second knock while still recovering from this? How would you know when your brain has recovered completely?"*
- Encourages reflection: *"How do you feel about this graduated return to sport that the sports doctors and rugby doctors are advising these days?"*

Poor communication with the patient:
- Fails to undertake a reassuring systematic examination.
- Fails to discuss 'concussion'. Without this information, the patient is not empowered to amend their concerns and expectations.
- Is overly blasé or overly defensive. The assessment becomes a tick box exercise without the questions being woven into the consultation. The consultation becomes mechanical and lacks flow.

Background knowledge required for this case

http://bjsm.bmj.com/content/43/Suppl_1/i85.full.pdf

Relevant literature

For a podcast tutorial, listen to:
Tinyurl.com/CS3e-Tc3a

From **Consensus statement on concussion in sport: the 4th International Conference on Concussion in Sport held in Zurich, November 2012.** *Br J Sports Med* 2013; **47:** 250–8 (doi:10.1136/bjsports-2013-092313)

Suspect concussion if the patient has one or more:
- Symptoms – somatic (e.g. headache), cognitive (e.g. feeling as if in a fog) and/or emotional symptoms (e.g. lability)
- physical signs (e.g. loss of consciousness, amnesia)
- behavioural changes (e.g. irritability)
- cognitive impairment (e.g. slowed reaction times)
- sleep disturbance (e.g. insomnia).

A player with diagnosed concussion should not be allowed to return to play on the day of injury.

Graduated return to play protocol

Rehabilitation stage	Functional exercise at each stage of rehabilitation	Objective of each stage
1. No activity	Symptom limited physical and cognitive rest	Recovery
2. Light aerobic exercise	Walking, swimming or stationary cycling keeping intensity <70% maximum permitted heart rate No resistance training	Increase HR
3. Sport-specific exercise	Skating drills in ice hockey, running drills in soccer. No head impact activities	Add movement
4. Non-contact training drills	Progression to more complex training drills, e.g. passing drills in football and ice hockey May start progressive resistance training	Exercise, coordination and cognitive load
5. Full-contact practice	Following medical clearance, participation in normal training activities	Restore confidence and assess functional skills by coaching staff
6. Return to play	Normal game play	

Teaching case 4 – Adult woman

Information for the doctor

Name	Anya Nedev
Age	36
Past medical history	Type 1 diabetes
	10 years ago recurrent depression
	3 years ago LLETZ for CIN 3
	1 year ago urticaria with Prozac
Current medication	Venlafaxine 75 mg twice daily
	Levemir Penfill injections 100 units/ml
	NovoRapid Penfill cartridges 100 units/ml
	Novo pens 3 and 4: 1–60 units
	Glucose oral gel 40%
	GlucaGen Hypokit injection 1 mg
	Test strips
	Ketone strips
BMI	25.6
BP	117/60

Information for the patient

You are 36 year old Anya Nedev, married for 3 years and planning a pregnancy. Your diabetologist recently advised how the insulin nurses would support you if you became pregnant. She also advised that you speak to your GP about coming off venlafaxine before you conceive.

Your opening statement is *"I've come to ask for your advice about using my venlafaxine in pregnancy."*

Information to reveal if asked

General information about yourself:
- You are a librarian at a local public school. You want to explore your treatment options to gain an understanding of risk. The diabetic consultant said that she thought it may be best to stop the venlafaxine before conceiving but as this was not her area of expertise, you may want to chat to your GP.
- You are not keen on stopping the venlafaxine because when you tried 5 years ago, you became very tearful, cried easily, lost control easily, felt panicked and had

difficulty leaving the house. However, you want a healthy baby and if the tablets are dangerous, then you'd like to know what your options are.

- You are happily married. You thoroughly enjoy your job and plan to return to full-time work after maternity leave.

Further details about your condition:

- You are aware that at age 36, your chances of conceiving are reducing with time, so you are concerned about how long it would take to come off the venlafaxine.
- You currently use barrier contraception.

Your ideas:

How dangerous is venlafaxine in pregnancy? If it is not very dangerous, you'd prefer to stay on the drug or drop to a lower dose.

Your concerns:

If you came off the venlafaxine and waited to see what happened to your mood, this may take too long and you may not have sufficient time for this. You want to start trying for a baby as soon as possible.

Your expectations:

You want the doctor's advice on the safety on venlafaxine as soon as possible. While it would be nice to get a consultant psychiatrist's opinion, you don't want to wait months for an appointment.

Medical history

You manage your diabetes well and do not have any complications.

Social history

Neither you nor your husband have children and you very much want to be parents. There have not been any specific problems at work.

Information to reveal if examined

You are currently not anxious or depressed.

Suggested approach to the consultation

Targeted history taking:

- When did Anya see the consultant and what was discussed? You have not received a copy of the hospital letter as yet.
- How many episodes of depression did she suffer? Were they related to life events? Did she become unwell quickly? Was she unwell for a long time before the medication became effective? When she was ill, how did this affect her family, friends, job and money? Was she able to tell that she was getting unwell?

- Does she have good support?
- Does she have a healthy lifestyle (balanced diet, minimal alcohol and no smoking, regular exercise, good sleep)? Is she taking folic acid?
- What does she understand by risk to the baby from venlafaxine? (picture the worst case on medication)
- What does she understand as risk to the baby of an untreated depression? Picture the worst case without medication. At her worst, how would she rate her ability to care for herself and the baby?
- How likely is she, if symptoms recur, to use alcohol or drugs instead to cope? How likely is low mood to affect her bonding?
- Picture the best case off medication.
- Picture the best case on medication.

Targeted examination:

- Examination is not required in this case.

Clinical management:

- Address the patient's ideas about risk to the pregnancy from venlafaxine. Inform her that in principle, no decision is completely free of all risks. There is a risk to the mother and baby from taking a medication in pregnancy. There is the risk of getting ill again from stopping a medication. Even if no medication is taken in pregnancy, up to 1 in 25 babies are born with a major problem (background risk).
- Fulfil her expectations for timely advice. Could you telephone or email a psychiatrist or pharmacist for advice?
- Once you have the information, you can help her to understand it but ultimately, she will need to make an informed decision.

Interpersonal skills:

Good communication with the patient:
- Demonstrates respect for autonomy, by helping the patient understand the issues so that she can make an informed decision.
- Demonstrates respect for diabetologist's advice. *"I'm so glad the diabetologist advised you to come to see me about this issue. It was also important that you didn't just stop your medication suddenly."*
- Shows responsiveness to the patient's preferences, feelings and expectations for further information on the risk of venlafaxine on pregnancy, the risk of relapse without medication, the possibility of reducing dose or changing medication.
- Communicates the relevant information in a manner that is understandable to the patient, without slipping into jargon and without patronising the patient.
Therefore, it results in addressing the patient's expectations appropriately.

Background knowledge required for this case

- Over 3000 pregnant women taking venlafaxine have been studied. In these studies women who took venlafaxine in early pregnancy were no more likely to have a baby with a birth defect than women who didn't.
- There has been one study which was designed to look for possible links between venlafaxine use in pregnancy and specific birth defects. It found a possible link between venlafaxine use in early pregnancy and heart defects in the baby. Venlafaxine is similar to selective serotonin reuptake inhibitors (SSRIs). Several studies investigating whether use of SSRIs in the first trimester of pregnancy might slightly increase the chance of the baby having a heart defect have produced mixed results. A link between venlafaxine or SSRI use in pregnancy and heart defects in the baby has therefore not been confirmed.
- One study also showed possible links with cleft palate, limb defects, gastroschisis and hypospadias. Because these results were from a single study, further research is needed to assess whether taking venlafaxine in pregnancy might increase the chance of certain specific birth defects in the baby.
- Three small studies that compared miscarriage rates between women taking venlafaxine and women not taking this medicine suggested that miscarriage may be more common in women taking venlafaxine, although a fourth study did not agree with this finding.
- There are a number of case reports of babies exposed to venlafaxine in late pregnancy who showed symptoms of neonatal withdrawal after delivery.
- There is currently very little information on whether use of venlafaxine in pregnancy increases the risk of persistent pulmonary hypertension of the newborn (PPHN). The only study to investigate this was very small and did not have enough women taking venlafaxine in pregnancy to be certain that the risk of PPHN is not increased.
- A single study has provided no proof that use of venlafaxine in pregnancy affects a child's intelligence or behaviour. More studies into the rates of behavioural and learning problems in children exposed to venlafaxine in the womb are required before we can say whether there may be any effects.

BUMPS (best use of medicines in pregnancy: www.medicinesinpregnancy.org) is a service provided by the UK Teratology Information Service (UKTIS). UKTIS is a not-for-profit organisation funded by Public Health England on behalf of the UK Health Departments. UKTIS (previously the National Teratology Information Service, NTIS) has been providing scientific information to healthcare providers since 1983 on the effects that use of medicines, recreational drugs and chemicals during pregnancy may have on the unborn baby. It has a good Patient Information Leaflet on venlafaxine in pregnancy: tinyurl.com/CS3e-Tc4a (*takes you to* www.medicinesinpregnancy.org/Medicine--pregnancy/Venlafaxine/)

Teaching case 5 – Adult woman

Information for the doctor

Name:	Ashmita Rai	
Age:	41	
Past medical history:	Three years ago	Rotator cuff syndrome
	Five years ago	Recurrent UTIs

The medical record of her **last consultation** by her GP (three weeks ago) reads:

"Had numerous investigations over many years including attempted egg harvesting. Notes from previous GP practice still not arrived – just registered here. She is hoping to meet with fertility consultant (private) to discuss why they were unable to harvest any eggs for freezing. 2nd husband. Both have undergone various tests."

Information for the patient

You are 41 year old Ashmita Rai. You finally called the Private Fertility Clinic you and your husband consulted 18 months ago to arrange a follow-up meeting, which you attended yesterday. You put off the meeting because you suspected bad news and it was confirmed yesterday when the fertility specialist told you that you will not be able to have children. You could consider egg donation or adoption, both of which you have not been able to get your head around as yet. You are deeply upset by the news that you will never be a mother.

Your opening statement is *"I'm so sorry to trouble you doctor but I just can't face going in to work at the moment"*.

Information to reveal if asked

General information about yourself, including occupation:
- You have been married to your current husband, Sanjay, for four years. Sanjay does not have any children. Your ex-husband now has 2 children with his new partner.
- You do 30 hours per week of computer-work (admin), including book-keeping, for an airport-based company, but most of your work can be done from home, with meetings at the airport. The commute is a nightmare. You have worked for this company for four years and like the work. A new HR person was hired three months ago and she has introduced efficiency measures, including asking for 'sick notes' from home-based workers.

Further details about your condition and circumstances that you reveal if directly asked:

- You are devastated by the news of not being able to have children of your own. You were unable to sleep. The fertility doctor's voice keeps playing in your head.
- You have a headache with muzziness, are sweating, and you feel generally weak with muscle ache. You can't stop thinking about not being able to have children. You don't want to talk to your husband (or anybody) about it at the moment. You feel numb and 'in shock'. You want to lie in bed and pull the duvet over your head.
- You are usually fit and healthy. You have not asked for a 'sick note' before.

Your ideas about what is happening to you:
- You think that you are in shock. You occasionally think the clinic made a mistake and maybe you should get a second opinion but deep down, you think you are clutching at straws. You need some time and space to pull yourself together.

Your concerns:
- You are worried about being a disappointment to yourself and your husband. You have 'failed'. Your dreams of children and how you imagined your future are smashed. This is very personal and you are concerned about what is written on the 'sick note'. You prefer the wording to be "complications from gynaecology treatment".

Your expectations of the consultation and of treatment:
- You want to be signed off for two weeks. You may consider medication for sleep but you are not keen on 'addictive' tablets. You do not want to be referred to a counsellor. The Fertility clinic offered you counselling and you made an appointment to see someone in 4 weeks (earliest available session).

Information to reveal when examined

You look upset and tearful. You are feeling hopeless; lacking in energy; tired; have no appetite; feel that you let yourself and your husband down and have trouble concentrating. You do not have thoughts of DSH.

Suggested approach to the consultation

Targeted history taking:

- What are Mrs Rai's symptoms? Are there physical symptoms, such as pain or palpitations? What are her feelings (detachment, disbelief, bitterness, loneliness, feeling dazed)?
- What are her thoughts on the news she has been given? What is the image going through her head when she recalls being told she is unable to have children? What sense has she made of the discussion?
- What is she doing; for example, is she able to function and complete activities of daily living? How clearly is she thinking? How safe is she? Any thoughts of self-harm?

- How severe are her symptoms? What are the worst symptoms? What would she like help with; for example, help with the intrusive thoughts disturbing sleep?
- The doctor obtains sufficient information to assess her distress, her ability to cope, and her current support networks.
- What is work like?
- What does she think is a reasonable amount of time off?
- What does she know about self-certification for illness and Fit notes?

Targeted examination:

- A brief mental health examination is required.

Clinical management:

- Address the patient's ideas – she believes she is in 'shock'; that is, in significant emotional distress. This is an understandable and appropriate response to the bad news she received. It is important to allow time to 'process' the news. Offer support.
- Address the patient's concerns about being a 'failure'. Explore if the patient could offer an alternative viewpoint, such as having tried her best or played a good game but not having the power to determine the outcome.
- If providing a Fit note, negotiate what is written on it.
- Fulfil her expectations for support, by listening, being empathetic and by discussing a possible short prescription of anxiolytics, such as zopiclone. Signpost to local sources of support. Offer follow-up.
- Be sensitive in discussing the 'sick note', which could easily have been the stated reason for attending, whereas the actual presentation was to discuss her bad news and obtain support. Be informed by Department of Work and Pensions, *Getting the most out of your fit note: GP Guidance* (Jan 2014): tinyurl.com/CS3-Tc5a (*takes you to* www.gov.uk/...fit-note-gps-guidance.pdf)

Interpersonal skills:

Good communication and negotiation with the patient involves making the care of your patient your first concern.
- Take the time to understand the patient's situation. Empathise with her difficulties.
- Offer practical support, or signpost to it.
- Act honestly. It is also appropriate to listen to Mrs Rai and to empathise with her bad news. Getting thrown by the 'sick note' request, becoming suspicious, sarcastic or rude would be unprofessional. While you need to respect the patient's right to confidentiality, be careful and truthful on what you write on a Fit note or private letter as the sick note policy should apply equally to all patients.

Background knowledge required for this case

A Cognitive Behavioural Therapy (CBT) approach could be helpful in structuring this consultation.

Fenn K and Byrne M (2013) The key principles of cognitive behavioural therapy. *InnovAiT: Education and inspiration for general practice*, **6(9):** 579–85. Available at: tinyurl.com/CS3e-Tc5b (*takes you to* http://journals.sagepub.com/...)

> CBT is based on the cognitive model of mental illness, initially developed by Beck (1964). In its simplest form, the cognitive model 'hypothesises that people's emotions and behaviours are influenced by their perceptions of events. It is not a situation in and of itself that determines what people feel but rather the way in which they construe a situation' (Beck, 1964). In other words, how people feel is determined by the way in which they interpret situations rather than by the situations *per se*. For example, depressed patients are considered to be excessively negative in their interpretations of events (Beck, 1976).

Reproduced with permission from SAGE.

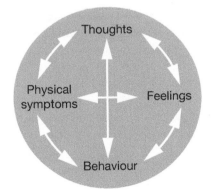

The hot-cross bun model of CBT formulation. From an idea attributed to Greenberger and Padesky (1995).

- Cognitions – an automatic thought (AT) is an interpretation of a situation (*"I am a failure"* rather than the situation itself (*"We cannot conceive naturally"*). People may be more aware of their emotional response (e.g. feeling numb or hopeless) to the situation rather than the AT thought itself.
- What could be the automatic thoughts running through Mrs Rai's head?
- What is her emotional response?
- What are her behaviours?
- The aim of a collaborative relationship in CBT is to examine (not directly challenge) the ATs.

One way of establishing rapport and empathy would be to use **empathetic reflections**:

- *"I can certainly understand how you might be feeling."*
- *"Your many attempts to become pregnant must feel overwhelming at times."*
- *"You sound like you want me to fix this issue with HR for you, which is understandable."*
- *"You sound exhausted by this."*
- *"It sounds like you don't quite know what you want to do next and need some thinking space."*

References

Beck AT (1976) *Cognitive Therapy and the Emotional Disorders*. New York: Penguin.
Beck JS (1964) *Cognitive Therapy: basics and beyond*. New York: Guilford Press.
Greenberger D and Padesky C (1995) *Mind Over Mood: a cognitive therapy treatment manual for clients*. New York: Guilford Press.

Relevant literature

Beck J (2011) *Cognitive Behavior Therapy: basics and beyond*, 2nd edition. New York: Guilford Press.
Beck Cognitive Behavior Therapy patient pamphlets. Available at: tinyurl.com/CS3e-Tc5c (*takes you to* www.beckinstitute.org/...)

Department of Work and Pensions (2014) ***Getting the most out of your fit note: GP Guidance***

Filling in the fit note
You can issue a fit note on the day that you assess your patient; or on any day afterwards.

The fit note should be completed as follows:
1. Write the date on which you assessed your patient. This can be via a face-to-face or telephone consultation; or consideration of a written report from another doctor or healthcare professional (for example nurses, occupational therapists, physiotherapists).
2. Describe the condition(s) that affect your patient's fitness for work. Give as accurate a diagnosis as possible, unless you think a precise diagnosis will damage your patient's wellbeing or position with their employer.
3. Tick 'not fit for work' OR 'may be fit for work taking account of the following advice'.
4. The comments box must be completed when you tick 'may be fit for work'. Completion is optional if you have ticked 'not fit for work'.
5. Indicate the period that your advice applies for. This may be the date that you expect your patient to have recovered by, or your judgement about an appropriate

time to review their fitness for work even if they are unlikely to have fully recovered.

6. Sign the fit note using ink.
7. Complete the date of statement. This is the date that you issue the fit note.

Your patient can go back to work at any point they feel able to, even if this is before their fit note expires. They do not need to come back to see you in order to do so, or get a new fit note. This is the case even if you have indicated that you need to assess them again.

How your patient will use their fit note

- If your patient is employed and you have indicated that that they are not fit for work, they can use the fit note to claim sick pay. Your patient should keep their original fit note and their employer may take a copy for their records.
- If your patient is employed and you have indicated that they may be fit for work, they should discuss your advice with their employer to see if there are changes which could support them to return to work (for example, changing their duties, adjusting work premises or providing special equipment). You do not need to suggest any of these changes – your advice is purely on the impact of your patient's health condition and it is up to your patient and their employer to discuss ways to accommodate it. If their employer cannot make any changes to accommodate your advice, the fit note is treated as if it stated that your patient was not fit for work. Your patient should not return to you for a new fit note stating this because they do not need one.
- If your patient is out of work, they can use a fit note to support a claim for health-related benefits or to show that they have been unable to fulfil certain benefit requirements. They can also use it in any discussions with prospective employers about supporting a health condition.

Teaching case 6 – Adult woman

Information for the doctor

Name	Evelyn (Evie) Thornton
Age	39
Social and family history	Married, one child
Past medical history	Not known – new patient
Current medication	Carbimazole 10 mg once daily
Information from new patient registration form	
Weight	46 kg
Height	157 cm
BMI	18.6
BP	106/64

Information for the patient

You are Evie Thornton, a 39 year old part-time saleswoman for a national clothing company. You were diagnosed with post-partum hyperthyroidism approximately 3 months ago after weight loss (1 stone), fatigue, itchy skin and heat intolerance. Your last GP started you on carbimazole 10 mg once daily. Your last T4 was 43 and she advised you to get monthly T4 measurements to check if you are on the correct dose. You are bottle-feeding.

You present to the doctor requesting a prescription of carbimazole and to arrange blood tests. Your opening statement is *"I need a prescription for my thyroid medication please. I brought my tablets with me"*.

Information to reveal if asked

General information about yourself:
- As a part-time employee newly transferred to the local office, a new mum with a 7 month old baby, and recently moved to the area, you are a bit stressed by all the changes. However, your mum lives nearby and helps you with childcare.
- Your relationship with your husband is 'fine'. After being made redundant, he found a new job, hence your move.
- You enjoy your work and would have liked to have had a longer maternity leave, but you need the income.

Further details about your condition:
- You have no side-effects from carbimazole. Since starting it, you gained the 1 stone and you are keen not to put on extra weight, having been slim all your life. You were warned your thyroid will 'burn out' and will become underactive, at which time you will need to take thyroxine replacement tablets.
- Prior to your diagnosis with hyperthyroidism, you were in good health and ran 3 miles four times per week. You are a non-smoker. You drink a glass of wine with most meals.
- Nobody in your family has thyroid disease.

Your ideas:
- You think your last GP was excellent. If she felt you needed monthly blood tests, then you expect the new GP to organise this.
- Your T4 came down quite quickly to 43 and your last GP advised that it will come down further with ongoing carbimazole 10 mg. You are happy with this dose and you are not experiencing any side-effects.

Your concerns:
- You are worried about not having been referred to see a consultant. Your last GP said as you would be moving to a new area imminently, it would be better to discuss referral with your new GP.

Your expectations:
- You expect to be given a repeat prescription for carbimazole.
- You expect a blood test for T4 levels, information on how you would be informed of the results and appropriate carbimazole or thyroid replacement tablet dosing.
- You expect a referral to the local hospital.

Information to reveal if examined

If the doctor asks to examine your thyroid gland, hand him/her a card saying "no goitre palpated. No bruit heard".

If the doctor asks to check your cardiovascular system, hand him/her a card saying "BP 110/68, pulse 86 regular".

Suggested approach to the consultation

Targeted history taking:

- Does Evie currently have any symptoms – fatigue, weight loss, palpitations, nervousness, irritability, heat intolerance?
- When does Evie take her medication? Is she compliant?
- Why was she put on this dose of carbimazole?
- Did she have other blood tests – TSH receptor antibodies or TPO antibodies or radioiodine uptake scans?

- What job does she do? Could Evie be anxious about her new job, etc.?
- What does Evie know about her condition?
- What are her expectations of this consultation: a prescription, further blood tests, a change in her medication, referral to an endocrinologist, time off work?
- What is her general health like and how is she managing her new job / child care?
- Does anyone in her family have thyroid problems / autoimmune disease and what has their experience of the illness been?

Targeted examination:

- A targeted physical examination of the thyroid is required to assess whether a goitre is present. See www.youtube.com/watch?v=JYb-io13fOA for a demonstration on how to examine the thyroid gland.

Clinical management:

- Explore Evie's understanding of an overactive thyroid – is this the thyrotoxic phase of post-partum thyroiditis (PPT) or Graves' disease presenting for first time in pregnancy? The thyrotoxic phase of PPT occurs between 1 and 6 months post-partum (most commonly at 3 months) and usually lasts only 1–2 months. Symptoms during the thyrotoxic phase of PPT tend to be milder than during hyperthyroidism due to Graves' disease. 95% of women with Graves' disease are TSH receptor antibody positive. In contrast to Graves' disease, PPT is characterised by decreased RAI uptake (measurement of ^{131}I uptake is contraindicated in lactating women) and are usually TPO-Ab positive.
- Discuss the significance of the negative examination findings.
- Her idea that blood tests are needed is valid. Discuss the need to request a few blood tests: TFT (TSH may be suppressed for months and therefore unreliable, so it is important to measure T4 and T3); TPO antibodies and TSH receptor antibodies (TSH-RAb).
- Discuss her concerns about not having seen an endocrinologist. Once blood tests are back (or obtained from her previous GP), and if TSH receptor antibodies are positive, the diagnosis of Graves' disease is made and referral to endocrinology (except for email advice) may not be needed. Graves' disease is confirmed by testing for tTSH-RAb, which have up to 98% sensitivity and 99% specificity for this condition.
- Address the patient's concerns and expectations: test TFT every 4–6 weeks and alter carbimazole dose according to T4. Once Evie is euthyroid, the dose of carbimazole is reduced until she is on the lowest amount necessary to maintain T4 and T3 within the normal range. Remission is usually achieved in 18–24 months, after which attempts may be made to cease medication.
- Explain how to take the medication. Encourage compliance with the medication. The British Thyroid Foundation provides a leaflet, *Your guide to antithyroid drug therapy to treat hyperthyroidism*, available at tinyurl.com/CS3e-Tc6a (*takes you to*

http://www.btf-thyroid.org/.../40-antithyroid-drug-therapy-guide, which may be helpful.

- Safety-net: advise Evie of how you intend to inform her of her blood results, carbimazole dosing (organise repeat prescriptions) and raise the next test request.

Interpersonal skills:

This case tests the doctor's ability to discuss with a patient her new diagnosis and plan for her ongoing care. The patient has a relatively good understanding of her condition, to which the doctor can add. The patient's agenda includes obtaining consultant advice but the GP could negotiate obtaining further testing to differentiate between PPT and Graves' within Primary Care. The skilful doctor reviews the issue systematically, negotiates the conflicting agendas and works in partnership with the patient.

The poor communicator is unable to devise a safe management plan: by requesting the wrong tests at the incorrect time intervals; by not being able to advise on medication dosing or simply by referring to endocrinology without advancing the patient's understanding.

Background knowledge required for this case

De Groot L, Abalovich M, Alexander EK, Amino N *et al.* (2012) Management of thyroid dysfunction during pregnancy and postpartum: an Endocrine Society clinical practice guideline. *Journal of Clinical Endocrinology and Metabolism*, **97**(8): 2543–65.

- PPT is the occurrence of thyrotoxicosis, hypothyroidism, or thyrotoxicosis followed by hypothyroidism in the first year post-partum in women who were without clinically evident thyroid disease before pregnancy.
- It is believed to be caused by an autoimmunity-induced discharge of preformed hormone from the thyroid. PPT occurs almost exclusively in women who are thyroid antibody positive. TPO-Ab positivity is the most useful marker for the prediction of post-partum thyroid dysfunction.
- The thyrotoxic phase of PPT occurs between 1 and 6 months post-partum (most commonly at 3 months) and usually lasts only 1–2 months.
- It is important to differentiate between the thyrotoxic phase of PPT and Graves' disease presenting *de novo* in the post-partum period.
- Symptoms during the thyrotoxic phase of PPT tend to be milder than during hyperthyroidism due to Graves' disease.
- Furthermore, 95% of women with Graves' disease are TSH receptor antibody positive.
- In contrast to Graves' disease, PPT is characterized by decreased RAI uptake (measurement of ^{131}I uptake is contraindicated in lactating women).

Being professional

Being professional is an important aspect of the therapeutic relationship. Being too close risks being too emotional and losing objectivity; being too distant places empathy at risk. Part of being professional is knowing one's limits and acting within one's capabilities.

The GMC states: "Good doctors make the care of their patients their first concern: they are competent, keep their knowledge and skills up to date, establish and maintain good relationships with patients and colleagues... are honest and trustworthy, and act with integrity and within the law....... Good doctors .... do their best to make sure all patients receive good care and treatment that will support them to live as well as possible, whatever their illness or disability."

This case was made deliberately difficult and it tests the professionalism of those doctors who lack the medical knowledge to advance the treatment plan beyond the patient's agenda. Doctors who pretend to know more than they do and attempt to 'bluff' their way through the scenario could be viewed as acting dishonestly, beyond their competence and not making patient care their first concern. This would be marked as a clear fail.

Teaching case 7 - Adult man

Information for the doctor

Name:	Herman de Groot
Age:	37
Past medical history:	12 years ago Type 1 diabetes 4 years ago Patello-femoral knee joint pain syndrome
Medication:	Levemir Penfill injections 100 units/ml NovoRapid Penfill cartridges 100 units/ml Novo pens 3 and 4: 1–60 units Glucose oral gel 40% GlucaGen Hypokit injection 1 mg Test strips Ketone strips

Last consultation: Oct last year – seen by practice nurse.

Patient was diagnosed with type 1 diabetes 12 years ago. His diabetic control is good and his recent IFCC A_1C was 56.

Has had flu vaccination previously with no problems. Comes for flu vaccination today. Offered pneumococcal vaccination – accepted.

Patient is able to self-monitor his blood glucose and is well educated and motivated in diabetes self-care. Will telephone for advice if develops side-effects to vaccination.

Information for the patient

You are a 37 year old lecturer. You were diagnosed with type 1 diabetes after a sudden short illness 12 years ago, which prompted a medical discharge from the Army. You are proactive in optimising your blood sugar management. Over the past few months you have experienced more hypoglycaemic episodes, despite the medication and your weight remaining unchanged. Initially, you used to check your BMs 8–10 times per day but once medication and routine stabilised, you now check 4 times per day.

You are seeing the GP today because your last hypoglycaemic episode scared you. You gave yourself your insulin injection, put your pasta bake in the oven, but fell asleep in front of the TV. Your 10 year old son, who was staying over, roused you when you failed to respond to the oven timer as quickly as he did, but you were able to take your oral glucose, administer glucagon and restore your BG by eating your pasta meal.

Your opening statement is *"I've been having some low blood sugars recently and wondering if I should cut down my insulin?"*

Information to reveal if asked

General information about yourself:
- When first diagnosed, you were told yours was an unusual presentation at your age. The Army doctor sent you on a 2-week residential course, where you learnt how to match your carbohydrate requirements with exercise demands.
- You used to be physically very active. Now you exercise for 30 minutes 1–2 days per week.
- You can usually tell when your BG is dropping. When you experience this vague sensation, you test yourself. If your BM is < 4, you are able to treat yourself with dextrose tablets or glucose gel and you recover quickly.
- You are now a civilian Ministry of Defence employee and teach vehicle maintenance at a local Army base.

Further details about your condition:
- You have been experiencing an episode of hypoglycaemia every 1–2 weeks for the last few months, usually in the afternoons.
- During these episodes, you feel anxious and nauseated, a bit sweaty but cold in your fingers. When you test your BG, they can be anything from 2.5 to 4.5. You feel better once you eat. You have not brought your BG booklet with you.

Your ideas:
- You separated from your wife three months ago and moved into a flat. Initially you thought the stress was making you feel anxious and sweaty. Now you think it is diabetes, probably because your diet has changed. You buy lunch now, have more pre-prepared supermarket meals and your alcohol consumption has increased.

Your concerns:
- You do not want to have hypoglycaemia, especially now that you are living alone. You worry that if your son hadn't been there, the oven alarm may not have roused you from your snooze and perhaps you could have gone into a coma or died. However, you have always had 'tight' control and you do not want your HbA1c to increase.

Your expectations:
- You expect the GP to give advice on how much insulin to take and perhaps to refer you back to the hospital Diabetic Clinic or enrol you on a refresher Diabetes Course.

Information to reveal when examined

In the last month, your lowest blood glucose was 2.5 and highest was 14.5. If the doctor asks to examine your injection sites, hand over a picture from tinyurl.com/CS3e-Tc7a (*takes you to* www.nejm.org/doi/full/10.1056/NEJMicm1101527 t=article) or tinyurl.com/CS3e-Tc7b (*takes you to* www.ncbi.nlm.nih.gov/pmc/articles/PMC3743397/)

Suggested approach to the consultation

Targeted history taking:

- Did Herman experience hypoglycaemia? – did he have:
  - warning symptoms of altered mental status, sympathetic nervous system stimulation or gastrointestinal symptoms;
  - with BG concentrations ≤3.1 mmol/L when symptoms were present; and
  - reversal of symptoms when he took glucose?
- How frequent are the episodes? Is he alone during episodes? How often has he needed help from others, including paramedics? Has he sustained any injuries?
- Has his lifestyle changed recently? How has his separation affected his diet (content, portion, regularity); his exercise; alcohol intake; job; socialisation with friends; weight?
- Has his insulin regimen changed with regard to type of insulin, dose, frequency, and care of injection sites?
- What does he tend to do in the hours preceding a hypoglycaemic episode?

Targeted examination:

- Ask to review his BG booklet.
- Examine his injection sites.

Clinical management:

- Make a diagnosis of hypoglycaemia caused by lipohypertrophy, which is benign tumour-like swelling of fatty tissue at the injection site secondary to lipogenic effect of insulin. Advise rotation of insulin injection sites, but use 10% less insulin at the new site. He may require advice about the type of needle and insulin, so referral to Diabetic Clinic may also be needed. Explain that depending on the severity of lipohypertrophy, the area may take some time to recover (from weeks to several months or longer).
- Educate Herman about how to avoid hypoglycaemic episodes, recognise the warning symptoms and start treatment early to reverse hypoglycaemia.
- It may be useful for Herman to diarise his symptoms, his activity levels, details of meals and timing and dosage of anti-diabetic medications, to try to identify reversible causes which can be addressed.

- Ask Herman to take BG readings using a quality-checked meter – do fasting, before meals, before bedtime, before driving, and occasionally at night (if hypoglycaemia at night is a problem). Correlate these readings with symptoms to assess if he is symptomatic at lowered BG readings, or symptomatic at high BM readings (the latter is possibly a sign of poor BG control).
- Check that he knows not to substantially delay treatment of hypoglycaemia by doing a BG if he is convinced that his symptoms indicate hypoglycaemia.
- Request blood tests: renal and liver function and HbA1c.
- Organise review with BG and symptom diary whilst awaiting Diabetic Clinic review.
- Discuss hypoglycaemia and fitness to drive.

Interpersonal skills:

This case tests the doctor's ability to assess why a stable condition has deteriorated (lipohypertrophy and lifestyle changes). The GP gives advice on rotating injection sites and making lifestyle changes. The patient, though currently reasonably well educated about hypoglycaemia, may need reminding about recognition of symptoms and the need for immediate treatment with oral glucose or IM glucagon, and is advised on how to access emergency care if required; the doctor safety-nets appropriately. The GP does not shy away from a discussion on fitness to drive.

Additional information

Driving

It is the responsibility of the driving licence holder to notify the Driver and Vehicle Licensing Agency (DVLA) of their medical condition.

Remind diabetic drivers to have a supply of a fast-acting carbohydrate in the vehicle and avoid driving if their meal is delayed.

Check their blood glucose level just before they start the journey, and then every two hours during the journey. If the blood glucose is low, they should:
- Stop the car in a safe place, switch off the engine, and move from the driver's seat.
- Eat or drink something containing a fast-acting carbohydrate.
- Wait until 45 minutes after the blood glucose has returned to normal before continuing the journey.
- Take regular meals, snacks, and rest periods on long journeys, and always avoid alcohol.
- Carry diabetes identification in case of injury in a road traffic collision.
- Take particular care during changes of insulin regimens, changes of lifestyle, exercise, and travel.

For Group 1 entitlement (to drive a car or motorcycle)

The person must satisfy the following criteria:

- Has adequate awareness of hypoglycaemia.
- Must not have had more than one episode of hypoglycaemia requiring the assistance of another person in the preceding 12 months.
- There should be appropriate blood glucose monitoring, defined as no more than 2 hours before the start of the first journey and every 2 hours while driving.
- Must not be regarded as a likely source of danger to the public while driving.
- The visual standards for acuity and visual fields must be met.

If the medical standards are met, a 1-, 2- or 3-year licence will be issued.

For Group 2 entitlement (to drive large vehicles like lorries and buses)

The person must satisfy the following criteria:

- Has full awareness of hypoglycaemia.
- No episode of hypoglycaemia requiring the assistance of another person has occurred in the preceding 12 months.
- Regularly monitors blood glucose at least twice daily (including on days when not driving), and at times relevant to driving (no more than 2 hours before the start of the first journey and every 2 hours while driving), using a blood glucose meter with a memory function to measure and record blood glucose levels.
- More frequent testing may be required if for any reason there is a greater risk of hypoglycaemia, for example after physical activity or altered meal routine.
- At an annual examination by an independent consultant diabetologist, the last 3 months of blood glucose readings must be available.
- Uses a modern blood glucose meter which has a memory chip to store 3 months of reading.
- Must demonstrate an understanding of the risks of hypoglycaemia.
- There are no other debarring complications of diabetes, such as a visual field defect.

If the medical standards are met, a 1-year licence will be issued.

Potential pitfalls

- **Beta-blockers** may blunt the sympathetic drive, which is responsible for the early signs of hypoglycaemia, so patients may not complain of symptoms until their blood glucose becomes dangerously low. A lack of hypoglycaemia awareness can have significant impact on a patient's lifestyle and ability to drive.
- Diabetics with **autonomic neuropathy** (often as a complication of long-term diabetes) can also lose the ability to sense typical hypoglycaemic symptoms.
- Conversely, patients with poor glycaemic control often complain of sympathetic symptoms early when their blood glucose is normal or high. They do not require glucose so should monitor their capillary blood glucose levels when they get these symptoms.

References

See Appendix D in the Driver and Vehicle Licensing Agency (DVLA) 2016 document *Assessing fitness to drive – a guide for medical professionals* for more information: tinyurl.com/CS3e-Tc7c (*takes you to* www.gov.uk/...)

NICE (2015) *Type 1 diabetes in adults: diagnosis and management* (NICE guideline NG17). Available at www.nice.org.uk.

Teaching case 8 – Adult woman

Information for the doctor

Name	Julia Pulaski
Age	51
Social and family history	Married, three children
Past medical history	Hypercholesterolaemia for three years
Current medication	Atorvastatin 10 mg daily
Blood tests	*Blood tests done 8 months ago*
Plasma fasting glucose	5.4 mmol/L (3.65–5.5)
Fasting cholesterol	5.1 mmol/L
Fasting HDL cholesterol	1.4 mmol/L (0.8–1.8)
Total cholesterol:HDL	3.6
Alkaline phosphatase	164 IU/L (95–280)
Total bilirubin	17 µmol/L (3–17)
Albumin	39 g/L (35–50)
Creatinine level	102 µmol/L (70–150)
BMI	26
BP	138/82

Information for the patient

You are Julia Pulaski, a 51 year old PA to a software executive, who has called the GP to discuss your 'dizziness'. You want to know if it is serious, how quickly it will pass, and if you can 'get something to help' with your symptoms. You are scared by how suddenly the 'dizziness' developed and how you feel dizzy when you move your head.

You call the doctor to discuss your symptoms and to see if you need a home visit for an examination.

Information to reveal if asked

Further details about your condition:

- Your dizziness started this morning when you rolled over to your left to get out of bed. The room felt like it was spinning and you felt so 'sea-sick' and nauseated that you quickly lay back down in bed. Moving brings on the spinning / unbalanced sensation so you are lying on your bed.

- The dizziness comes and goes. At its worst, it feels like it lasts 5 minutes and is accompanied by nausea. In between these attacks, you feel like your head is in cotton wool / foggy and your thinking is not clear.
- When you sit or lie still in one position, whether on your back or on your side, you don't get the rolling / tumbling sensation. When you move, you get it but not always. If questioned in detail, it is sudden fast movements to the left (rolling over to get out of bed; turning to use the towel; turning to get a mug from the bedside cabinet) that brings on the attack. Not all attacks are equally severe; the initial ones are the worst.

Your ideas:
- You think that you may be having a stroke, but you are trying hard not to panic. Maybe it just something silly and short-lived or easily cured.

Your concerns:
- You are worried about what it is, how long it's going to last and how it's going to affect your ability to work / do household chores / drive.
- When you called in sick, your boss asked if you'd be well enough for the business trip next week (3-hour train journey for each leg).

Your expectations:
- You want a diagnosis and information. If you need an examination, you request a home visit.

General information about yourself:
- Your husband has gone into work. He left you a vomit bowl and some apple juice. You don't feel you can leave the house today.
- You do not smoke and drink 3 large glasses of wine per week.

Information to reveal if examined

This is a telephone consultation and no examination is done.

Suggested approach to the consultation

Targeted history taking:

- What are Julia's current symptoms? Once you have asked open questions (*"Describe the dizziness"*) and closed questions (*"Are you experiencing ringing in your ears / a feeling of fullness in the ear / difficulty hearing?"*) you could summarise the problem back to her – *"So, in summary, you are experiencing episodes of dizziness, a tumbling / spinning sensation, lasting about 5 minutes, provoked mainly by fast movements, especially when turning to the left, eased by lying or keeping still, associated with nausea and accompanied by a foggy head in between attacks."*
- Excludes red flags – for tumour (unremitting vertigo with severe nausea and vomiting and no relief in any position) and stroke (face, arms, speech affected).

- What does she think are causing these symptoms?
- What treatments has she tried already?
- How are her symptoms affecting her home and work life?
- What are her expectations of this consultation: a telephone discussion, an examination either by coming to the surgery or a home visit, time off work, medication, advice, or signposting to patient information leaflets?

Targeted examination:

- Not done. This is a telephone consultation.

Clinical management:

- On the basis of probability, the doctor makes a diagnosis of benign paroxysmal positional vertigo (BPPV). Discuss the diagnosis and natural history in jargon-free language.
- Discuss that examination involves doing a Dix–Hallpike manoeuvre: www.youtube.com/watch?v=8RYB2QlO1N4 . If the test is positive, it confirms the diagnosis of BPPV but if negative, it only tells you that the problem in the ear is not active at the moment the test is being done.
- Address the patient's ideas: she believes that her dizziness may be a presentation of stroke. Discuss risk factors and presentation of (cerebellar) stroke and how her presentation differs.
- Address the patient's concerns about prognosis, impact on ADL (including driving and train journeys) and effective treatment. Options include treatment of nausea; it is best to avoid vestibular sedatives which only provide minimal relief, are not curative and can cause grogginess. Discuss Epley's manoeuvre – www.youtube.com/watch?v=jBzID5nVQjk. The dizziness with BPPV is variable; in some patients it is provoked by train journeys. She can drive unless dizziness remains disabling or is precipitated by driving.
- Address the patient's expectations: she believes that she needs a home visit. The initial symptoms are very scary and patients often overestimate (probably from fear) the duration of dizziness, so 20 seconds may feel like 5 minutes. Now that she is provided with some information, does she want to reconsider home visit request? Negotiate a management plan. Consider 'prescribing' Epley's (if there is someone in surgery who can perform the manoeuvre) or refer to audiology clinic. The cure rate after two sessions can be as high as 95%.
- Safety-net: follow-up should be arranged for performing Dix–Hallpike test; performing Epley's; reviewing if there is no response to Epley's or if the patient opts for watch and wait, if dizziness continues for >4 weeks.

Interpersonal skills:

This case tests how skilfully doctors explore a frightening symptom and through systematic questioning and adequate information-sharing, reframe the patient's health beliefs. She is empowered to change her ideas, be reassured about her concerns and shift her expectations. After the discussion about the diagnosis and options, it is important to check her understanding, ask if she has questions and signpost to relevant information. A useful question could be *"Having discussed our options, what would you like me to organise for you?"*

Background information required for this case

Treatment options:
- Watchful waiting to see whether symptoms settle without treatment.
- Offer Epley's manoeuvre. Ideally this should be done at the first presentation in primary care if the expertise and time are available. Symptoms may improve shortly after treatment, but full recovery can take days to a couple of weeks. If symptoms do not settle after 1 week and the diagnosis of BPPV is not in doubt, advise the person to return and consider repeating the Epley's manoeuvre.
- Consider suggesting Brandt–Daroff exercises which the person can do at home, particularly if the Epley's manoeuvre cannot be performed immediately or is inappropriate.
- Symptomatic drug treatment is not usually helpful for people with BPPV.

Advise the patient to return for follow-up in 4 weeks if symptoms have not resolved, in case BPPV has been incorrectly diagnosed.

Useful resource with video clips

tinyurl.com/CS3e-Tc8a (*takes you to* www1.imperial.ac.uk/...otology/mabdandv/

Teaching case 9 – Adult man

Information for the doctor

Name	Russell Dunn	
Age	33	
Social and family history	Self-employed fitter and joiner; single	
Past medical history	4 years ago	Anxiety with depression
	6 years ago	Anxiety with depression
	11 years ago	Asthma
Current medication	Clenil CFC-free inhaler 100 mcg/actuation 2 puffs twice daily	
	Salbutamol CFC-free inhaler 100 mcg/puff as required	
From 6 months ago	Never smoked	
	1–2 units alcohol per week	
BMI	27	
BP	136/85	
Peak flow (best recorded)	550	

Information for the patient

You are Russell Dunn, a 33 year old self-employed fitter and joiner with a tight chest and wheeze on the back of a cold which started last week. You have used your inhalers but the chest remains tight. Your cough is productive of yellowish sputum. You still feel warm, tired and have muscle ache with your cold. You are concerned that the infection spread to your chest and think you may need antibiotics.

Your opening statement is, *"I know you doctors don't like giving antibiotics but my chest is bad doctor."*

Information to reveal if asked

General information about yourself:
- You are self-employed but you don't always have sufficient money for your inhalers. You tell the practice nurse that your asthma is better than it actually is. No one has questioned you about using 3 brown inhalers and 6 blue inhalers in the last year.
- You have episodes of 'chestiness' most years but things are OK if you avoid sport, outdoor activities and smoky environments.

Further details about your condition:
- If specifically asked, you had a blocked / runny nose, sore throat, headache and tiredness for 7 days. Then you started to cough and your chest felt tight. Cough was worse at night and productive.
- You are currently fitting a new shop. It is dusty at work but the room is well ventilated and you wear a mask when sawing / planing. Your symptoms were as bad over the weekend (away from work) as when you are at work.
- You were once admitted overnight to hospital (A&E ward) for treatment of asthma age 21.

Your ideas:
- You think the infection has gone to your chest. You expect a prescription for antibiotics. You are not allergic to anything.

Your concerns:
- You are worried about missing work. You want the building contractor to use you again in his other projects.

Your expectations:
- You expect to get an examination and medication for your chest. You won't be surprised that this may be asthma and you can afford the inhalers at present. You find the blue one works quickly so you always keep a blue one handy but you do not have a brown one at present. You are reluctant to take time off to return for reviews.

Information to reveal if examined

You are talking normally and can finish your sentences.
Peak flow 350, 340, 360
O_2 sats 97%
RR 20
Pulse 83, BP 142/84
Temp 36.8°C
Widespread expiratory wheeze; no crackles

Suggested approach to the consultation

Targeted history taking:

- What are Russell's current symptoms? What medication has he tried and what was the response?
- How are his symptoms affecting him, especially with regard to sleep and his ability to work safely with tools?
- What does Russell think is causing his cough and tight chest? Has he done a peak flow at home? How brittle (and severe) is his asthma?

- Has Russell used antibiotics (or inhalers) for these symptoms in the past and have they helped?
- What does Russell think would be a good compromise with respect to management: salbutamol via a spacer or nebuliser (by the practice nurse or at home), oral prednisolone 40–50 mg for 5 days, a written action plan and information on how to access emergency or out of hours care, delayed script for antibiotics (to be used only if evidence of chest infection develops) and primary care review within 1–2 days?

Targeted examination:

The targeted physical examination should include PF, oxygen sats, respiratory rate and pulse.

Clinical management:

- Address Russell's ideas: build on his idea that the infection is responsible for his cough and tight chest. However, this is probably not due to direct spread of infection but rather that it has triggered an excess immune response.
- Address his concerns: that the illness will affect work. Russell is not describing conditions at work (dust, cold) that aggravate his symptoms, nor is he describing exposure to irritant or sensitising substances.
- Address his expectations: of a prescription. He needs treatment for a moderate exacerbation, which if ignored or inadequately treated, or if he has a poor response to treatment, may need hospital admission.
- Discuss the need to take this presentation of asthma exacerbation seriously. Negotiate and develop a shared plan.
- Discuss follow-up.
- Provide a written personal asthma action plan (PAAP) – tinyurl.com/CS3e-Tc9a (*takes you to* www.asthma.org.uk/.../adult-asthma-action-plan.pdf).

Interpersonal skills:

This case tests the doctor's ability to:
- assess the physical symptoms to grade severity of the asthma attack and also to undertake a *holistic* assessment (asthma and work)
- negotiate a management plan and timely review
- prescribe appropriately, in line with current UK guidance.

Good communication with the patient:
- Explores and acknowledges the reasons for the patient's attendance – to resolve chest symptoms quickly.
- Appreciates that Russell may have an underlying fear about job security, finances and the ability to afford medication and time off work.

- Explores his expectations of treatment. By discussing that most asthma deaths occur in patients not using adequate doses of inhaled or oral steroids, and in whom there is a severe underuse of PAAPs, Russell is empowered to make decisions on medication and follow-up.
- Achieves a shared understanding, and negotiates an appropriate and acceptable management plan.

Poor communication with the patient:
- Fails to appreciate the financial concerns driving Russell's denial about the severity of his asthma.
- Is prescriptive and fails to adapt the asthma guideline to the individual patient.

Background knowledge required for this case

SIGN (2016) *British guideline on the management of asthma.*
www.sign.ac.uk/pdf/QRG153.pdf

It is important to get a clear picture of what has been happening with the patient to accurately assess what the problem may be but not to delay treatment whilst gathering an extensive history. As per the BTS/SIGN asthma guidelines (2016), raised pulse and respiratory rate are indicators of acute asthma. Peak flow below 75% of best or predicted indicates a moderate attack; below 50% indicates a severe attack and below 33% a life-threatening emergency, so it is important to always attempt to measure this as a marker of severity. It is also difficult to gauge response to treatment without measuring these parameters at base line.

Difficulty with speech, reduced consciousness and use of accessory muscles (in children) are all indicators of severe asthma. It is better to use pulse oximetry to assess hypoxia as visual assessment of cyanosis is not reliable and cyanosis may not be apparent until saturations are as low as 67%.

Immediate treatment with high dose bronchodilators is essential. A spacer and MDI have been shown to be effective in all but life-threatening incidences. It is important to give each dose separately and not all together, to ensure maximum benefit; by doing this the dose can be tailored to the individual response. If a nebuliser is used it should ideally be oxygen driven but this needs flow rates of 6–8 L, often not available from a domestic cylinder, and the dose would be 5 mg salbutamol.

The earlier in an attack oral steroids can be given, the better the outcome. Treatment should be continued daily for at least 5 days or until recovery. If improvement occurs it is essential to ensure that the family and patient know how to respond to any further deterioration and have instructions on what to do. Review within 24 hours is required to ensure that response to treatment has been maintained and to review the circumstances leading up to the attack, to try to avoid future occurrences.

If, after one hour, response to treatment is limited, this is a poor prognostic sign therefore immediate transfer to hospital by ambulance is required. An ambulance is a safe environment with access to resuscitation equipment.

Teaching case 10 – Adult man

Information for the doctor

Name	Paul Walker
Age	22
Social and family history	Single, no children, fireman
Past medical history	Calf pain 6 months ago – had physiotherapy
	Closed fracture R little finger 5 years ago
	Greenstick fracture L radius 12 years ago
Current medication	None
Clinical values	*From 6 months ago*
BMI	25
BP	122/76

Information for the patient

You are Paul Walker, a 22 year old fireman, who has come to discuss a slightly embarrassing problem. Over the last month, both breasts have slowly increased in size and are tender to touch. You do not like the appearance and have become self-conscious.

Your opening statement on presentation today is *"I've come about an embarrassing problem doctor"*.

Information to reveal if asked

General information about yourself:
- You joined the fire service a year ago. One of your colleagues competes at body building and you, an active sportsman (ice skating and hockey) started some gym work with him.
- Six months ago, he offered you 'designer' drugs to build muscle, which he said he used safely for years. After researching it on the internet, you decided to take a course of 4 cycles, comprising tablets and injections. In the middle of the 2nd cycle, you developed breast tenderness which stopped when the cycle ended. In your 3rd cycle, you have developed breast swelling and tenderness. Your colleague told you to see your GP to get tamoxifen to prevent this 'side-effect'. He told you not to tell the GP about your drug use because doctors wouldn't prescribe tamoxifen if they think you abuse drugs.
- You do not have any growth or testicular problems. You did not find any testicular lumps when you last checked.

- You do not smoke and you rarely drink. You have a very healthy low carbohydrate, high protein diet.

Your ideas:
- You think the body-building drugs produced the breast enlargement and that tamoxifen will help to shrink them back to their normal appearance.

Your concerns:
- You are worried about the doctor becoming suspicious. You plan to stick to your story of breast enlargement with tenderness, which is affecting your ability to move fire-fighting equipment (when the hoses, etc. rub across your chest, it is painful).

Your expectations:
- You expect to get a prescription for tamoxifen, which you came across in your internet research.

Medical history

You are fit and healthy.

Information to reveal if examined

If the doctor asks to do a breast examination, hand him or her a card saying 'bilateral 3 cm firm glandular swellings around the nipple areola complex' and a picture from www.gynecomastia.org/photo-galleries

If the doctor asks to do a testicular examination, hand him or her a card saying 'normal size testes; no masses'.

Suggested approach to the consultation

Targeted history taking:

- What are Paul's symptoms? Describe the rate of growth. As regards breast tenderness, elicit intensity, duration, aggravating and relieving factors.
- If thinking about gynaecomastia, what could have caused an imbalance in the free oestrogen to free androgen ratio, resulting in this condition? Are there any medical conditions (hyperthyroidism, liver cirrhosis / renal insufficiency, testicular tumours) that could be causing this problem? Is he taking any medication, or using drugs / alcohol / herbs? Has the patient experienced symptoms of hypogonadism – impotence, decreased libido and strength?
- Are there any red flags – a stony hard, immobile, non-tender swelling; skin dimpling; nipple retraction; nipple discharge or lumps in the armpit to suggest breast cancer? Is there a testicular lump?

- How do symptoms impact on his work and home life? Is he socialising, in a relationship, maintaining good mental health? Assess how body image, self-esteem and sexual function have been affected?
- Does he have any ideas about how this condition could be treated?
- What are his concerns? Is he worried about cancer? Is he embarrassed about his appearance and what is the impact on his mood and confidence?
- What are his expectations: did he have any specific medication in mind; did he want to discuss scans, did he want a referral?
- What is his general health like? In younger men, it is important to explore use of illicit drugs and body-building supplements. Anabolic steroids, even 'designer pro-hormones', can suppress the body's endogenous testosterone. Some athletes take human chorionic gonadotrophin (hCG) to overcome the hypogonadism, but hCG can increase oestrogen levels, which worsens the gynaecomastia.

Targeted examination:

Check the breasts and testes and assess secondary sexual characteristics.

Clinical management:

- Empathise with Paul: you can see how his breast swelling is embarrassing him, and you recognise that it is important to treat this condition.
- Explain why it is important to understand the condition (the glandular tissue proliferates, then fibroses / thickens). If anything is driving proliferation of breast tissue (such as some types of BP medication), the best thing to do is stop the drug. Tamoxifen (unlicensed use, mainly for breast pain) can be tried for 3–9 months, but may be effective when used in the proliferative (not fibrotic) phase. Side-effects include DVT, loss of libido, bone pain, neurocognitive deficits, leg cramps and ocular events, some of which, if they develop, impact on his career as a fireman.
- Discuss the options: it may be useful to make a general statement such as *"If I were seeing a patient whose breast enlargement were the side-effect of medication I had prescribed, the first thing I would do would be to stop the tablet. I would not continue to use the medication and treat breast enlargement with tamoxifen – that tends not to work. In someone in'whom we didn't know what was causing the breast enlargement, I'd do some blood tests to look for a cause. If I did prescribe tamoxifen, I would speak to the patient very carefully about how effective it could be, and the harms it could cause. As a fireman, if you developed problems with your eyes or concentration, that could have consequences for your career."*
- Establish a plan: offer to do blood tests (9am testosterone, LFTs, TSH, U&Es).
- Address the patient's ideas: agree that gynaecomastia needs treatment but the correct treatment needs careful consideration. Medical options – tamoxifen, danazol, clomiphene have potential harms and surgical options (usually for the fibrotic stage) are rarely funded on the NHS.
- Address the patient's concerns: that the breast pain affects his work. As a fireman, does he have access to Occupational Health services?

- Address his expectations: discuss the need to investigate the problem further before considering a prescription for tamoxifen. Discuss how prescriptions need to be evidence-based, in line with *BNF* advice.
- Confirm his understanding of what gynaecomastia is and his treatment options.
- Safety-net: arrange review after Paul has his blood tests.

Interpersonal skills:

This case tests the doctor's ability to recognise presentations with a hidden agenda. If the doctor is unable to create a trusting relationship in which he or she can give the patient sensible information (to counterbalance the information his body-building colleague is giving him), then the opportunity to positively influence his lifestyle choices is lost.

When doctors become emotional about certain presentations (for example, if they become overtly suspicious, annoyed, fearful), then their ability to communicate clearly may be affected. In this case, if information is given in a balanced manner and in jargon-free language, the patient's understanding of the benefits and risks of tamoxifen is altered. By the end of the discussion, the patient should feel sufficiently informed that he can make his own decision about which option is best for him.

Good communication with the patient:
- Empathises with his 'embarrassing' appearance.
- Excludes red flags – breast and testicular cancer.
- Responds to the patient's request for tamoxifen in a safe and professional manner.
- Provides explanations that are relevant and understandable to the patient.

Poor communication with the patient:
- Makes assumptions about the patient, or is overly confrontational.
- Does not inform the patient of his options. The doctor prescribes or refuses to prescribe tamoxifen without much discussion.
- Instructs the patient on lifestyle choices.
- Uses inappropriate or technical language.

Background knowledge required for this case

Thiruchelvam P *et al.* (2016) Gynaecomastia. *BMJ*, 354:i4833
tinyurl.com/CS3eTc10a (*takes you to* www.bmj.com/...)
Reproduced with permission from BMJ Publishing Group Ltd.

The history is typically of slow breast enlargement, which is either bilateral or unilateral. Size can vary. Breast tenderness and pain around the nipple area are common symptoms, owing to proliferation of glandular tissue. Consider malignancy and refer urgently to a breast specialist any man who presents with a suspicious breast mass.

When examining, calculate body mass index and assess secondary sexual characteristics. Examine the breasts by palpating all areas of the breast tissue (including the nipple) and examine the axilla. Compare and note if enlargement is unilateral or bilateral. Palpable, firm, glandular tissue (>2 cm) in a concentric glandular mass around the nipple areola complex is most consistent with gynaecomastia.

Tamoxifen is the most widely used medical treatment, but it is not licensed for gynaecomastia. Response rates of up to 95% have been reported with tamoxifen (trials of between 2 and 12 month treatment durations). Tamoxifen has been shown to improve breast pain and is more effective when gynaecomastia is less than 4 cm. Trial doses vary and there is no clear guidance on treatment dose or duration. There are no good data to support treatment beyond nine months, and effects are usually seen after three months.

Drugs known to cause gynaecomastia:
- Anti-androgens – bicalutamide, flutamide, finasteride, dutasteride (AA)
- Antihypertensive – spironolactone (AA)
- Antiretrovirals – protease inhibitors (saquinavir, indinavir, nelfinavir, ritonavir, lopinavir), reverse transcriptase inhibitors (stavudine, zidovudine, lamivudine) (UM)
- Environmental exposures – phenothrin (antiparasitical)
- Exogenous hormones – oestrogens (EP), prednisone (male teenagers), human chorionic gonadotrophin (E)
- Gastrointestinal drugs – H2 histamine receptor blockers (cimetidine) (AA), proton pump inhibitors (e.g. omeprazole) (AA)
- Analgesics – opioid drugs (RA)
- Antifungals – ketoconazole (prolonged oral use) (AA)
- Antihypertensives – calcium channel blockers (amlodipine, diltiazem, felodipine, nifedipine, verapamil) (UM)
- Antipsychotics (first generation) – haloperidol (IP), olanzapine, paliperidone (high doses), risperidone (high doses), ziprasidone
- Antiretrovirals – efavirenz (UM)
- Chemotherapy drugs – methotrexate, alkylating agents, e.g. cyclophosphamide, melphalan (AA); carmustine, etoposide, cytarabine, bleomycin, cisplatin (AA), vincristine (AA), procarbazine
- Exogenous hormones – androgens (misuse by athletes) (EP)
- Cardiovascular drugs – phytoestrogens (soya-based products, high quantity) (EP)
- Recreational / illicit substances – marijuana, amphetamines (UM), heroin (UM), methadone (UM), alcohol
- Herbals – lavender, tea tree oil, dong quai (female ginseng), *Tribulus terrestris*, soy protein (300 mg/day), *Urtica dioica* (common nettle)

AA = anti-androgenic; RA = reduced androgens; E = oestrogenic; IAM = increased androgen metabolism; ISHBG = increased concentration of sex hormone binding globulin; IP = increased prolactin; UM = unknown mechanism.

Further reading

tinyurl.com/CS3e-Tc10b (*takes you to* www.nhs.uk/.../breast-reduction-male.aspx)
tinyurl.com/CS3e-Tc10c (*takes you to* http://baaps.org.uk/procedures/gynecomastia)
tinyurl.com/CS3e-Tc10d (*takes you to* www.england.nhs.uk/.../N-SC006.pdf)

Teaching case 11 – Adult man

Information for the doctor

Name	Benjamin Gilbert
Date of birth (Age)	68
Social and Family History	Divorced, with two children who live nearby.
Past medical history	Hypertension for 13 years
	Intermittent lower back pain
Current medication	Bendroflumethiazide 2.5 mg once daily × 28
	Atenolol 50 mg once daily × 28
	Ibuprofen 400 mg thrice daily or as required × 100
	Paracetamol 1 g four times daily or as required × 100
Private prescription	Sildenafil 100 mg as directed × 4
Blood tests	*Blood tests done 3 months ago*
BP	148/90
Urea and electrolytes	within normal range
Liver function tests	within normal range
Serum cholesterol	6.5
Cholesterol/HDL ratio	6.0
Fasting triglycerides	1.8
Fasting glucose	5.4
Current smoker	10 cigarettes per day for 35 years

Information for the patient

You are Benjamin Gilbert, a 68 year old retired plumber, who experienced severe chest pain last night (within the last 12 hours). It woke you up from sleep. You were about to call the ambulance when it eased after 20 minutes. You thought it would be best to get it checked out this morning.

Your opening statement is *"I'm worried about my heart, doctor. I had some chest pain last night but it could have been the pork pie I had for tea."*

Information to reveal if asked

General information about yourself, including occupation:
- You are a retired plumber, but you still occasionally help your son out with local jobs.
- You are divorced. You have been in a relationship with a new partner for the last eight months.

Further details about your condition:
- If specifically asked about the chest pain, it is a heavy weight in the centre of your chest (8/10) that woke you up from sleep. You thought to get a drink of water but didn't feel you could move during the pain. Despite lying quite still in bed, you were sweaty. You are not currently in pain but you feel quite drained.
- If asked about where the pain was, it was in your central chest. You did not have arm or jaw heaviness or pain.
- You wonder if it could be indigestion but you did not have any acid reflux, even with taking ibuprofen, and you don't usually get heartburn except after heavy meals with lots of alcohol, such as at Christmas dinner. It wasn't the same type of pain.
- You do not have any chest pain or shortness of breath now.
- You have not had chest pain or heart problems in the past. Your BP is usually OK, and you take your medication regularly.
- You are usually fit and healthy. You continue to smoke 10 cigarettes per day.

Your ideas about the illness, your treatment preferences, your coping skills and beliefs about healthcare:
- You suspect you may have had a heart attack but you are hoping the doctor will check you over and tell you that you are fine.

Your concerns about the illness, treatments, prognosis, length of illness, effects on work and role:
- You are worried that this may turn out to be a heart attack or something quite serious.

Your expectations of the consultation and of treatment:
- You expect to be examined and reassured. You don't want to get alarmed over nothing.

Information to reveal if examined

Pulse 88 regular
BP 156/96
Respiratory rate 20
Oxygen saturation 96%

Suggested approach to the consultation

Targeted history taking:

- Take a detailed history of Benjamin's symptoms:
  - chest – onset, intensity, aggravating and relieving factors, radiation, associated symptoms
  - risk factors for cardiac chest pain
  - complications such as heart failure, palpitations or small recurrences of chest pain.
- Explore Benjamin's ideas about why the pain may or may not be a heart attack or indigestion.
- He stated his fear about a 'heart attack' at the outset. Explore these concerns and discuss what a 'heart attack' is and what you need to do to rule it out.
- Explore his expectations – he expects an examination, and you need to assess pulse, BP, respiratory rate, oxygen sats, ECG and advise on the urgency of ordering investigations. As the chest pain occurred in the last 12 hours, he will need referral as an emergency if the 12 lead ECG is abnormal or if you cannot do an ECG at the surgery. If the ECG is normal, he will still need referral for urgent same day assessment.

Targeted examination:

- Perform a BP, pulse, respiratory rate and oxygen sats.
- Organise an ECG – the patient does NOT hand you a ECG.

Clinical management:

- Organise a 12-lead ECG.
- Give aspirin 300 mg.
- Discuss a possible diagnosis of acute coronary syndrome (ACS).
- Discuss the treatment options – as he is currently pain free, he does not need GTN or diamorphine.
- Address Benjamin's ideas: this chest pain is different in nature to the indigestion he has previously experienced. As a hypertensive smoker, with new onset chest pain at rest, lasting longer than 15 minutes and associated with sweating, this could be ACS. In the absence of breathlessness and an altered level of consciousness, he does not appear to have life-threatening complications.
- Address the patient's concerns about a heart attack. *"I think we need the results of the ECG and other blood tests, which the hospital needs to arrange for you, before we can rule out a heart attack. What do you think?"*
- After organising an ECG, refer to the hospital.
- Confirm his understanding of ACS and provide sufficient information about the condition and what he should expect in terms of investigation and treatment from the hospital.

- Arrange suitable GP follow-up after his cardiac assessment.

Interpersonal skills:

This case tests the doctor's ability to explore a presenting problem more deeply, eliciting the presence of 'red flags' resulting in the diagnosis of cardiac chest pain / ACS. It also tests the doctor's ability to prioritise treatment agendas: referral to hospital within 12 hours of cardiac chest pain takes precedence.

Good communication with the patient:
- Use of open and closed questions to explore the chest pain: *"Tell me what happened with the pain last night. Where was it? How long did it last? On a scale of 1 to 10, how severe was it?"*
- Makes statements to widen the patient's agenda: *"I agree with you that we need to rule out a heart attack, or acute coronary syndrome as the hospital doctors will call it. Do you know anyone who had hospital tests for a heart attack? Well this is what the hospital will need to do for you..."*
- Builds trust through reflective listening: *"It sounds like you want to believe it's indigestion but it's good that you didn't bury your head in the sand about heart problems. Let's get the results of the ECG and arrange for some hospital blood tests. The blood tests have to be done within 10 to 12 hours from when the chest pain started. How does that plan sound?"*
- Encourages reflection: *"Look, you came in thinking I'll just examine you and here I am sending you for an urgent ECG and hospital blood tests. How do you feel about this?"*

Poor communication with the patient:
- Fails to explore the red flag – cardiac sounding chest pain occurring within the last 12 hours.
- Fails to discuss what ACS is and explain why urgent diagnosis and treatment is needed. Without this information, the patient is not empowered to amend their concerns and expectations.

Background knowledge required for this case

NICE (2016) CG95. *Chest pain of recent onset.* tinyurl.com/CS3e-Tc11a (*takes you to* www.nice.org.uk/...) (see *Table 6* on p. 54)
Timmis A. (2015) Acute coronary syndromes. *BMJ*, 351.

Relevant literature

http://emedicine.medscape.com/article/1910735-overview

Definition of acute coronary syndrome:
Acute coronary syndrome (ACS) refers to a spectrum of clinical presentations ranging from those for ST-segment elevation myocardial infarction (STEMI) to presentations

found in non–ST-segment elevation myocardial infarction (NSTEMI) or in unstable angina. It is almost always associated with rupture of an atherosclerotic plaque and partial or complete thrombosis of the infarct-related artery.

Symptoms – patients with ACS may complain of:
- palpitations
- pain, which is usually described as pressure, squeezing, or a burning sensation across the central chest and which may radiate to the neck, shoulder, jaw, back, upper abdomen, or either arm
- exertional shortness of breath that resolves with pain or rest
- sweatiness, nausea or vomiting
- decreased exercise tolerance.

Signs or physical findings can range from normal to any of the following:
- Hypotension: indicates ventricular dysfunction due to myocardial ischaemia, myocardial infarction (MI), or acute valvular dysfunction.
- Hypertension: may precipitate angina or reflect elevated catecholamine levels due to anxiety or to exogenous sympathomimetic stimulation.
- Sweatiness.
- Pulmonary oedema and other signs of left heart failure.
- Extracardiac vascular disease.
- Jugular venous distension.
- Cool, clammy skin and sweatiness in patients with cardiogenic shock.
- A third heart sound (S3) and, frequently, a fourth heart sound (S4).
- A systolic murmur related to dynamic obstruction of the left ventricular outflow tract.
- Rales on pulmonary examination (suggestive of left ventricular dysfunction or mitral regurgitation).

Potential complications include the following:
- Ischaemia: pulmonary oedema.
- Myocardial infarction: rupture of the papillary muscle, left ventricular free wall, and ventricular septum.

Teaching case 12 – Adult woman

Information for the doctor

Name:	Lyndsay Marsh	
Age:	45	
Past medical history	13 years ago	Non-insulin-dependent DM
	Five years ago	Knee pain
	Ex-smoker	
Current medication	Lisinopril 5 mg once daily	
	Gliclazide 80 mg twice daily	
	Ezetimibe 10 mg once daily	
Problems with medication	Developed severe pruritis on three different statins	
	Stopped Avandamet 2 mg + 1 g OD six years ago	
Social history	Married with one teenage son. Works in marketing.	
Blood tests	*Blood tests done 6 weeks ago*	
HbA1c	8.3 (4–6)	
Total cholesterol	5.2	
Urea and electrolytes	no abnormalities	
Liver function tests	no abnormalities	
FBC	no abnormalities	
TSH	2.5 (0.3–4.2)	
BP	132/89	
BMI	53 (height 168 cm, weight 150 kg)	
Urine dipstix	negative for blood and protein	

Practice nurse's consultation from last month:

The plan reads:

"Discussed not meeting BMI target but patient tells me she was discharged from MoreLife (had counselling), feels unable / unwilling to change current lifestyle and does not want bariatric surgery. Discussed not reaching HbA1c target and patient would like to discuss treatment options with GP – appointment made."

Information for the patient

You are 45 year old Lyndsay Marsh. You have been overweight for years and you have given up on weight loss programmes. You have come to see the GP to discuss what to do about your increasing HbA1c. The nurse told you it is possible to set individual targets and you could stick to your current medication, or you could take more tablets or you could go onto insulin. You don't want to use insulin. Your aunt put on a lot of weight when she was put onto insulin and you would rather not self-inject. You do not have a problem with using injectables but think taking tablets would be less hassle.

Your opening statement is *"I've come to talk to you about my HbA1c".*

Information to reveal if asked

General information about yourself, including occupation:
You work in marketing, doing 24 hours per week of mainly office-based work, which you enjoy. You are a keen blogger and tweeter. You blog and tweet about food, local food events, recipes, restaurants and farming practices. You have tried to lose weight but failed. You accepted that you are a 'fat person' and a 'foodie'. You do not want to talk about lifestyle changes; you want to discuss medication.

Further details about your condition and circumstances that you reveal if directly asked:
- You are intrigued by the nurse's statement that you don't have to reach an HbA1c target of 7.5 and that the doctor has revised the target for you. What does this mean?
- You want to know what tablets you can take.
- You are usually fit and healthy.

Your ideas about what is happening to you:
You think that your diabetes is OK. You don't feel unwell and you don't get side-effects from the medication you are currently taking. You prefer taking tablets for diabetes.

Your concerns:
You are worried about not reaching the target HbA1c of 7.5g%. What would happen in the long term if you accepted an HbA1c of 8 or 9? Is the NHS trying to save money by not prescribing more tablets? You worry about weight gain on insulin.

Your expectations of the consultation and of treatment:
You want to discuss treatment options and would prefer to get a prescription for a third tablet, as least on a trial basis.

Suggested approach to the consultation

Targeted history taking:

- How does Mrs Marsh feel about her recent HbA1c? What does she already know about her treatment options?
- What are her thoughts on accepting an HbA1c of 8.3g%, given that lower targets (of 8 and 8.5) are set for frail or end-stage patients or those with cognitive impairment? Also if 1000 diabetics were treated over 5 years to achieve a drop in HbA1c of 0.9%, then eight CV events would be prevented.
- If she is not keen on insulin, she could be offered several tablets. What does she know about gliptans, pioglitazone (she used Avandamet in the past) or gliflozins?
- Has she experienced hypoglycaemia on gliclazide? Would she be able to recognise and treat a possible hypoglycaemic episode?
- What is her work and family life like at present and how would she manage a change in medication?

Targeted examination:

- An examination is not required.

Clinical management:

- Address the patient's ideas – she worries about weight gain with insulin and this is a possibility. She used Avandamet in the past and did not experience any side-effects, so adding on a pioglitazone may be useful in increasing her sensitivity to circulating insulin but she could gain 3–4 kg in weight. While she does not have contraindications to gliptans (heart failure) or gliflozins (renal impairment), they carry the risk of pancreatitis and recurrent UTIs/thrush respectively. Gliptans are weight neutral and gliflozins could give some weight loss.
- Address the patient's concerns about accepting a higher HbA1c, weight gain with insulin and financially-sensitive prescribing. Some of the newer drugs may be more expensive but there is no good evidence to say that any class of drugs is better at lowering HbA1c than any other. Choice of a new hypoglycaemic agent should be guided by whether it increases her risk of hypoglycaemia; the possible effect on her weight; possible contraindications / cautions; her current renal function and cost-effectiveness.
- After weighing up pros and cons, fulfil her expectations for a third tablet, and advise she should halve her gliclazide when starting the new drug, to reduce the risk of hypoglycaemia. Offer follow-up HbA1c in 2–6 months, and increase gliclazide dose as needed.

Interpersonal skills:

Good communication with the patient:
- Sets priorities – after checking that she remains unmotivated (despite significant previous time and resource investment) to lose weight, the challenge is to move on to the HbA1c target.
- In dealing with the HbA1c, the doctor negotiates acceptable, individualised HbA1c targets and provides sufficient information on the options available to enable patient choice.

The doctor:
- adopts a person-centred approach and works in partnership with the patient – gives her the options, discusses with her the risks and benefits of each option, and allows her to reach her own decisions.
- reconciles the health needs of the individual patient and the health needs of the community, balancing these with available resources – tactfully discusses medication costs, and how this, as well as risk of hypos, effect on weight gain, etc., guide local protocols and prescribing habits.

Background knowledge required for this case

Pages 8–11 of the following resource are very useful: tinyurl.com/CS3e-Tc12a (*takes you to* www.nice.org.uk/...patient-decision-aid-2187281197)

NICE (2015) guideline NG28. *Type 2 diabetes in adults: management.* www.nice.org.uk/guidance/ng28

- Involve adults with type 2 diabetes in decisions about their individual HbA1c target.
- Aim to avoid adverse effects (including hypoglycaemia) or efforts to achieve their target which impair their quality of life.
- Involve adults with type 2 diabetes in decisions about their care, individualising this to take account of each person's preferences, comorbidities, risks from polypharmacy or tight glucose control, and life expectancy.
- Support adults to aim for an HbA1c target of 48 mmol/mol, rising to 53 mmol/mol as treatment intensifies.

Teaching case 13 – Teenage girl

Information for the doctor

Name	Nicola Bradshaw
Age	17
Social and family history	At college
Past medical history	R patello-femoral maltracking 3 years ago – had physiotherapy
	L shoulder pain 4 years ago – posture-related
	Asthma 4 years ago
Current medication	Salbutamol take 1 puff 20 minutes before exercising
	Qvar – take 1 puff twice daily
	Marvelon take 1 tablet for 21 days, then have a 7-day break
Clinical values	*last seen 3 months ago*
BP	112/72
Height	176 cm
Weight	72 kg
BMI	23
Spirometry	FEV_1 at 4.17 L (112% predicted)
	FVC 5.25 (125% predicted)

Information for the patient

You are Nicola Bradshaw, a 17 year old college student. Over the last 4 years, you have experienced episodes of shortness of breath, difficulty speaking, wheeze and upper chest tightness during rowing training and competitions. You were diagnosed as asthmatic and treated with a brown inhaler and a blue inhaler for 3 years.

Last week, when you undertook a high intensity ergometer session (involving very fast rowing), you became extremely short of breath, your throat and chest felt sore and tight and you wheezed. You had to stop rowing. Within 3 minutes of stopping, the symptoms disappeared. You thought you may be developing a cold, but when you felt well 3 days later, you tried the high intensity session again. Despite taking the blue inhaler 20 minutes before the session, exactly the same thing happened. You want a referral to the hospital to get 'properly checked out' and to get better medicines so you can row competitively.

You present to the doctor wishing to get something done about your exercise-induced wheeze. Your opening statement is *"I'm fed up with this asthma affecting my rowing"*.

Information to reveal if asked

General information about yourself:
- You compete at a high level in rowing. You may get a rowing scholarship for University.
- You are a relaxed person. You do not stress about competitions. You enjoy the team spirit and competing is good fun. Even if you don't win, you like going to races and you like keeping fit.

Further details about your condition:
- If specifically asked, you do not have chest pain, palpitations or childhood lung or heart conditions. You have not coughed up blood.
- Your wheeze starts during exercise, when you try to put in maximum effort. Your throat and lungs feel like they are closing up. Your wheeze gets really loud. Your coach calls you Monica (after Seles; a tennis player notorious for her habit of grunting or shrieking loudly when hitting shots) instead of Nicola, because of the sounds you make.
- You are very rarely ill. You do not have any long-term illnesses, nor do you smoke.

Your ideas:
- You think that you need better inhalers.

Your concerns:
- You are worried that people might think you have psychological hang-ups about competitions. These episodes occur when you are working hardest and come on during competitions, but also when you are training hard. They happen whether you are happy or down, relaxed or anxious.

Your expectations:
- You just want to be referred to a specialist, preferably someone with an interest in Sports.

Medical history

You are in good general health, currently using Marvelon for contraception and using your inhalers as the practice nurse showed you.

Social history

You are happy at school with a busy and full social life.

Information to reveal if examined

If the GP asks, you have a recording of your breathing that your coach made for you: www.youtube.com/watch?v=60nfsxsaGmU (play this sound to the GP).

Suggested approach to the consultation

Targeted history taking:

- What are Nicola's current symptoms?
- For how long has she had these symptoms?
- Does she have red flags: exercise-induced chest pain or palpitations, or haemoptysis?
- Does Nicola have a history of atopy or allergy; family history of atopy; cough coming on within seconds of the peak exercise and settling within a few minutes of rest; chest symptoms not affected by inhalers; throat and upper airway tightness; speech problems or symptoms precipitated by exercise / cold air / strong odours / stress? Does she have indigestion / reflux or symptoms of post-nasal drip?
- How do symptoms affect her home and school life?
- Does she have a cough that disturbs sleep?
- What treatments has she tried already?
- Does she have any childhood illnesses or does she take any medication to enhance her sporting performance?
- What does she think is causing her illness?
- Does she have any particular concerns?
- What are her expectations of this consultation: an examination and reassurance, further investigation, alternative medication, a note for a competition?
- What is her general health like?

Targeted examination:

- A targeted examination of the neck and chest is required.

Clinical management:

- Discuss the difficulty in diagnosing the cause of exercise-induced wheeze because most of the symptoms and signs occur during strenuous exercise and assessment during the resting state is unlikely to be helpful.
- Explain that selfie mobile phone video recordings may be informative.
- Discuss the possibility of this being exercise-induced laryngeal obstruction (EILO). The diagnosis involves referral to ENT for a continuous laryngoscopy exercise (CLE) test.
- Address the patient's ideas: she believes she needs a better inhaler. The best treatment for EILO has yet to be determined. However, it is advisable to avoid laryngeal irritants (e.g. caffeine, untreated reflux, cigarette smoke), and to have regular fluid intake. To reduce alarming symptoms during peak training, Nicola could take a deep sniff, or breathe in through the nostrils and out through pursed lips. Once the diagnosis is made, Nicola may need referral to language therapists or physiotherapists to teach breathing and laryngeal control techniques. Surgical intervention has also been associated with good outcome.

- Address the patient's concerns: she is worried about being labelled as having psychological problems. While EILO may be precipitated by emotional stresses (such as competitions), it is thought that in EILO, the laryngeal aperture narrows at peak exercise, typically secondary to an 'in-folding' of the supraglottic structures. This may be followed by a degree of vocal cord closure, which increases turbulence and creates the typical symptoms of wheeze, shortness of breath, cough, and laryngeal irritability with a propensity to cough.
- Address the patient's expectations: she wants a referral, which is warranted. Refer to ENT for CLE, but getting good recordings of her wheeze and providing up-to-date resting and post-exercise spirometry or peak flow measurements may be useful to exclude asthma / exercise-induced bronchoconstriction.
- If you discuss medication, talk about the risks and benefits of rationalising inhaler use, bearing in mind that EILO can coexist with exercise-induced bronchoconstriction.

Interpersonal skills:

Good communication with the patient:
- Responds to her concerns about her symptoms being mistaken for competition stress. Discuss the original diagnosis (of exercise-induced asthma) needing review. It could be EILO, EILO coexisting with asthma or EILO being triggered by stress, but we don't have sufficient data as yet to make a firm diagnosis.
- Discusses the possibility of this being EILO in simple language, discusses how the diagnosis is made, and explains effective treatments briefly.
- Acts in an open and non-judgmental manner – in re-opening the diagnostic reasoning, is careful not to criticise colleagues who may not have considered alternative diagnoses and stuck to the diagnosis of EIB.

Poor communication with the patient:
- Does not work through the diagnostic sieve to review the diagnosis.
- Does not inquire sufficiently about the patient's niggling concern about being labelled as having 'competition stress'.
- Fails to safety-net with advice on what to do if she develops severe symptoms again while training.

Background knowledge required for this case

Hall A. *et al.* (2016) Exercise-induced laryngeal obstruction; a common and overlooked cause of exertional breathlessness. *Br. J. Gen. Pract.*, **66:** 490–1.

Unexplained breathlessness and cough are often attributed to the diagnosis of exercise-induced bronchoconstriction (EIB), and yet it is now recognised that exertional dyspnoea in athletes is frequently explained by the development of a transient obstruction, occurring at the level of the larynx. This condition, termed exercise-induced laryngeal obstruction (EILO), typically occurs during intense, competitive bouts of exercise and can explain why 'asthma-type' symptoms appear refractory to inhaled therapy.

The reason some athletes develop EILO is currently unclear. Several mechanisms have been postulated to explain development of EILO, and it is likely that laryngeal closure occurs as the result of a combination of factors.

In women, differences in the structure of the larynx may predispose them to develop EILO. An aspect of psychological stress arising from intense competitive environments may also play a role in the development of laryngeal dysfunction, and treatment with relaxation therapy should be considered.

www.ncbi.nlm.nih.gov/pmc/articles/PMC4933616/

www.youtube.com/watch?v=BAqj4b-AsnM

Learning consultation skills for COT and CSA

The aim of this section of the book is to encourage readers to practise patient consultations in preparation for COT and CSA. The reader is required to work out the necessary questions and conduct a 'consultation'.

Each of the 20 cases comprises the following sections.
- '*Summary of the patient*', including any recent test results – the basic background you need.
- '*Tasks for the doctor*' – what you are expected to establish in the consultation.
- '*More about the patient*' – more about the patient's background and presentation; this section can be used by a study partner to allow them to act as the 'patient'.
- '*Approach to be taken*' – this explains what the examiners are assessing with the case and provides a model answer.
- '*Test your theoretical knowledge*' – a short series of single answer multiple choice questions to test how well you understand current clinical practice; answers are provided at the end of the book.
- Each case ends with suggestions for further reading.

There are two ways to use this section of the book.
1. Ideally, you will work through the cases with a study partner, with one of you assuming the role of 'patient' and the other the role of 'doctor'.
    - The 'patient' reads the first two pages of the case, comprising the *Summary of the patient* and *More about the patient* sections – this allows them to understand the expectations of the patient so they can then answer the doctor's questions.
    - The 'doctor' should read only the first page comprising the *Summary of the patient* and should then conduct a consultation with the patient with a view to:
        A. gathering data to get to the nub of the problem
        B. managing the clinical problem
        C. demonstrating their interpersonal skills

2. Working alone, read through the first page and then note down the questions you would wish to ask in the consultation, referring to the *More about the patient* section as necessary. You may wish to use a COT *pro forma* for your answers.

COT *pro forma*[1]

A. Data gathering, examination and clinical assessment skills

1. Define the clinical problem:
- What questions do you ask to clarify why the patient has presented today?
- How would you explore the patient's ideas, concerns, expectations and health beliefs?

2. Perform an appropriate physical or mental examination
- What is the appropriate targeted physical or mental state examination?
- Can you perform the examination slickly and sensitively using appropriate medical equipment?

B. Clinical management skills

3. Make an appropriate working diagnosis
- On the basis of probability, what is your working diagnosis?

4. Explain the problem to the patient using appropriate language
- How would you explain the diagnosis to the patient?
- Is your explanation jargon-free, well organised and logical?
- Does it address the patient's concerns and expectations?

5. Provide holistic care and use resources effectively
- Was your management plan informed by national or local guidelines?
- Have you referred appropriately?

6. Prescribe appropriately
- Have you considered drug interactions or discussed side effects?
- Did you check the patient's understanding of the medication?

7. Specify the conditions and interval for follow-up
- Have you safety netted appropriately?

---

1   Adapted from a COT *pro forma* developed by Dr David Chadwick, Springfield Surgery, Oxfordshire.

C. Interpersonal skills: know and treat this patient

8. Achieve rapport
- Have you demonstrated active listening, sensitivity, and empathy?
- Have you used the patient's ideas and beliefs in explanations?
- Have you addressed the patient's specific concerns and expectations?

9. Give the patient the opportunity to be involved in significant management decisions
- Have you involved the patient in decisions?
- Have you negotiated, offered various treatment options or encouraged autonomy and opinions?

Long case 1 – Menopausal symptoms

Brief to the doctor

Mrs JS is a 51 year old woman who presents for treatment of her hot flushes. She used HRT tablets 2 years ago for peri-menopausal flushing and stopped 3 months ago after developing PV bleeding. Her hysteroscopy 1 month ago was negative. Having discontinued with the HRT 3 months ago, the flushes have recurred.

Patient summary

Name	JS
Date of birth (Age)	51
Social and Family History	Married, two children
Past medical history	Hysteroscopy (1 month ago) – no pathology
	Postmenopausal bleeding on HRT (3 months ago)
	Hip pain (1 year ago)
	Menopausal symptoms (flushing) for 2 years
Current medication	Ibuprofen 400 mg prn × 84
Blood tests	Tests were done 1 month ago (pre-hysteroscopy)
Plasma fasting glucose	5 mmol/l (3.65–5.5)
Fasting cholesterol	5 mmol/l
TSH	1.12
Hb	13.2 g/dl (13–17)
MCV	86 (83–105)
BMI	25.6
BP	117/60

Tasks for the doctor

In this case, the tasks are to:
- present Mrs JS with suitable treatment options for her hot flushes
- provide her with sufficient information to make an informed decision
- prescribe appropriately

Brief to the patient – more about the patient

1. Profile:

- Mrs JS a 51 year old woman
- married with 2 children, ages 18 and 15
- a paediatric out-patient nurse
- flushing is becoming a real nuisance: disturbs sleep, embarrasses her when it occurs at work and she feels tired
- she felt well on HRT but really disliked having a hysteroscopy for PMB so, if possible, would prefer not to restart HRT; she's read about soya and yams but is unaware of other treatment options

2. She is seeing the doctor today because:

- she has not had a period or any PV bleeding for 3 months; prior to this, she had withdrawal bleeds on the HRT
- she is not keen on hormone treatments or the Mirena coil; she does not have any other health problems and uses condoms for contraception
- she is now flushing more than three times per day every other day – her sleep is interrupted and she feels tired
- she is worried about her ability to maintain a calm and reassuring demeanour at work (paediatric OPD) if she continues to feel tired and irritable
- she expects the doctor to give her advice about complementary therapies, prescribe something or refer her to the Menopause Clinic – she wants an action plan for this problem and is not happy with a 'wait and see' policy
- she quickly grasps the medical information imparted and nods her head to indicate understanding of the treatment options
- if she feels coerced into choosing one option (such as HRT), she asks for a referral to the Menopause Clinic
- if the doctor laughs at her health beliefs, she challenges him on his views on complementary therapies
- if the doctor offers her SSRIs, at first she seems sceptical and asks if the doctor thinks she is depressed – she accepts this treatment after a discussion on its evidence, efficacy and safety

Approach to be taken

A. Data gathering, examination and clinical assessment skills

1. Define the clinical problem: clarify why the patient has presented today
The doctor:

- reads the patient summary provided prior to seeing Mrs JS
- detects Mrs JS's reluctance to restart HRT and her eagerness to explore alternative treatment options for her menopausal flushing
- asks open questions to explore the frequency, severity, impact of the flushing, and her specific concerns about HRT
- asks closed questions to ascertain the presence (or absence) of other menopausal symptoms, including periods
- excludes red flags, such as on-going PMB
- elicits how the problem affects Mrs JS at work (and at home)
- discovers Mrs JS's ideas regarding phytoestrogens
- discovers her concerns about further episodes of PMB on HRT
- discovers her expectations for further treatment, either conventional or complementary
- summarises the problem: *"Mrs JS, on stopping your HRT you have experienced flushes that interfere with your ability to work comfortably. You'd prefer not to take HRT and would like me to discuss alternative treatment options with you. Have I understood you correctly?"*

2. Perform an appropriate physical or mental examination

- In this case, neither a formal physical or mental state examination is required.

B. Clinical management skills

3. Make an appropriate working diagnosis
The doctor, based on the history and exclusion of 'red flags', makes a clinically sound working diagnosis – menopausal flushing.

4. Explain the problem to the patient using appropriate language
The doctor:

- explains that the menopausal flushing is a 'nuisance' problem rather than a 'serious health problem'
- agrees with Mrs JS that it should be treated to improve her quality of life
- discusses in jargon-free language the benefits and risks of HRT (IUS + oestrogen only HRT), transdermal HRT and phytoestrogens; may briefly mention second- and third-line alternatives such as escitalopram 10–20 mg or sertraline 50 mg, venlafaxine, gabapentin or clonidine, some of which can be initiated if recommended by the Menopause Clinic

- provides information in adequate chunks and checks understanding at each step
- uses the patient's ideas: phytoestrogens may be useful; isoflavones or black cohosh may relieve vasomotor symptoms. However, multiple preparations are available and their safety is uncertain. Different preparations may vary and interactions with other medicines have been reported.
- addresses the patient's concerns: further PMB on HRT may require investigation to exclude endometrial pathology, hence endometrial protection with an IUS and oestrogen-only HRT or SSRIs may be more acceptable to the patient
- addresses the patient's expectations – provides treatment options

5. *Provide holistic care and use resources effectively*
   The doctor:
   - may use or discuss complementary medicines, such as red clover and black cohosh
   - may use time as a therapeutic tool: if Mrs JS seems to have difficulty in making a decision regarding which treatment she would prefer, the doctor could offer a leaflet and provide a follow-up appointment
   - offers the treatment options and, if Mrs JS indicates that she would like to get her treatment sorted out today, helps her to choose the most appropriate therapy for her
   - demonstrates practice of evidence-based medicine – he discusses which treatment options have a good evidence base and are proven to be effective
   - is informed by national or local guidelines – tinyurl.com/CS3e-Lca (*takes you to* www.nice.org.uk/...managing-short-term-menopausal-symptoms)

6. *Prescribe appropriately*
   The doctor:
   - if prescribing transdermal HRT or SSRIs, chooses a cost-effective medication
   - prescribes the appropriate dose and number of tablets
   - discusses drug interactions and side effects
   - checks the patient's understanding of the medication

7. *Specify the conditions and interval for follow-up*
   The doctor:
   - safety-nets appropriately – when to consult again and why: *"Is it OK to meet again in a fortnight to check how you are getting on with this tablet? Obviously, if there are problems, I'd like to see you sooner."*

C. Interpersonal skills: know and treat this patient

8. *Achieve rapport*

   The doctor:

   - listens attentively to the patient's request for treatment and her concerns regarding PMB on HRT
   - displays empathy to the adverse effect flushing has on her confidence and comfort at work
   - is non-judgemental about the patient's health beliefs regarding complementary therapies
   - addresses the patient's specific concerns and expectations, for example, does not spend more time speaking about HRT and breast cancer when this is not the patient's specific concern; addresses her concern about the difficulty in differentiating between significant endometrial pathology and 'nuisance' break-through bleeding on HRT

9. *Give the patient the opportunity to be involved in significant management decisions*

   The doctor:

   - shares a raft of management options and involves the patient in decisions
   - negotiates with the patient which option may be better for her given her specific concern (HRT and BTB)
   - reassures the patient that the most effective treatment for peri-menopausal flushing is HRT (transdermal or HRT + Mirena are options) but phytoestrogens and SSRIs may be effective in reducing the frequency of flushing and are not, in this instance, being used to treat a psychological problem
   - encourages autonomy and opinions – with regard to complementary therapies, the doctor provides a balanced discussion regarding evidence, cost, etc., but refrains from making derogatory comments if he does not share these health beliefs

Debrief

Discuss how the doctor could, if needed, improve his performance. In particular, assess whether the doctor:

- empathised? If so, how?
- presented the patient with appropriate treatment options?
- explained the risks and benefits of treatments in simple language?

If the consultation over-ran:

- how could the history taking be shortened?
- how could the explanations be simplified?
- how could the doctor have expressed empathy and understanding? Comment on the doctor's non-verbal behaviour and his summarising.

Revising data gathering

Are there any existing medical records for the doctor to peruse before the patient consults?

- The doctor was given a patient summary prior to the patient's presentation.

What questions could the doctor ask to discover the patient's ideas, concerns, expectations and health beliefs?

- Ideas: *"I understand that you are not keen to restart HRT. Were there any other treatments you had in mind?"*
- Concerns: *"You don't seem keen on using SSRIs. Are there particular concerns you have about these tablets?"*
- Expectations: *"It seems to me the flushing is really interfering with your work and you want to discuss the risks and benefits of potential treatments. Shall we run through these options?"*
- Health beliefs: *"You know that HRT tablets may produce nuisance bleeding, but HRT (with a Mirena) is probably the most effective treatment for you. Alternatively, we could try SSRIs, which may be useful in reducing the frequency of menopausal flushing; it is not being used as an antidepressant here. In addition, there is no added risk of BTB with SSRIs, unlike HRT."*

Once the doctor has gathered sufficient information, how could he summarise the problem for the patient?

- *"Mrs JS, you have given me quite a lot of information. I'd like to summarise our discussion back to you so you can correct me if I've left out anything important."*
- *"You suffer from menopausal flushing. You have used HRT in the past but unfortunately developed BTB. You would like treatment of the flushing, but you would prefer to consider options other than HRT. In particular, you'd like to discuss the effectiveness and safety of natural oestrogens."*

Relevant literature

tinyurl.com/CS3e-Lca (*takes you to* www.nice.org.uk/...managing-short-term-menopausal-symptoms)

Long case 2 – Neck pain

Brief to the doctor

Mr AB is a 34 year old man who presents to your surgery with a 4 week history of neck pain that is getting progressively worse.

Patient summary

Name	AB
Date of birth (Age)	34
Social and family history	Single Lives with mother
Past medical history	Road traffic accident 17 years ago • Fracture of right femur and tibial plateau • Fracture of left ankle
Current medication	None

Investigations

	2 years ago:
BMI	34
BP	135/90
Urine	NAD on Multistix

Tasks for the doctor

In this case, the tasks are to:
- clarify the neck pain symptoms, identify causative factors (occupational history), perform an appropriate examination, formulate a diagnosis, and finally present Mr AB with appropriate management options and agree on a management plan
- undertake opportunistic screening in view of BMI and BP; explore his health beliefs about weight and identify factors that might motivate him to lose weight

Brief to the patient – more about the patient

1. Profile:

- AB is a 34 year old single man
- he works in the accounts department of a local business
- he has been getting neck pain for the past 4 weeks

2. He is seeing the doctor today because:

- the pain is getting worse; it is localised to the right side of his neck at the back and does not radiate and he has no sensory changes or weakness in the arms. The pain gets worse during the day at work. It does not disturb his sleep and is not present on waking. He does not get the pain at weekends, even though he spends a lot of the time looking after his mother who is 'crippled with arthritis'.
- he has started taking ibuprofen and paracetamol at work to ease the pain
- his work is sedentary, checking account details on the computer
- he would like to be referred for physiotherapy as he believes his pain is due to sitting in front of a computer all day; he is happy to be given postural advice or exercises. He does not like taking tablets as he feels they only mask the problem and he is worried that doing so will result in long term damage to his neck.

3. Additional information:

- If the doctor asks specifically:
  - he has been moved to a different area of the office following a restructuring of the company. His new desk is small and the screen is set to one side, so he has to twist to look at it. He has an adjustable chair, but it is broken and the height is no longer adjustable. He is reluctant to make a fuss, because so many people lost their jobs in the restructuring. He would really like a letter from the doctor to give to his occupational health nurse suggesting that his workplace may be contributing to, or even causing, his neck pain.
  - he has no past history of neck or back pain
  - he is worried that arthritis is hereditary and that he is getting arthritis in his neck
- If the doctor asks about his weight:
  - he has put on more weight since last weighed; his mother is also obese, as was his father until he died of a heart attack age 55 years
  - he snores, but has no daytime somnolence
  - he follows no special diet; his mother likes 'good old-fashioned English food'. He buys sandwiches or crisps for lunch and always has sweets and chocolate in his office drawer. He drinks 1–2 cans of beer in the evenings. He despises smoking.

- he knows he should lose weight, but finds it difficult to motivate himself, or to do it in isolation from his mother – he thinks eating is one of the few pleasures they both enjoy
- he is concerned about his future health, especially as his father died of heart disease; if the doctor advises him in unambiguous terms that losing weight would benefit his health, he would address the problem
- if the doctor examines him, his BMI is 36, BP 150/90; neck flexion and looking over his left shoulder is slightly reduced.

System	Findings
General	Central obesity. Waist 40 inches (102 cm) Posture – rounded shoulders, protruding head BMI 36
Cardiovascular	Pulse 78 SR HS 1+2 nil No evidence of cardiomegaly or cardiac decompensation BP 150/94
Endocrine	No evidence of thyroid disease Urine negative for glucose
Cervical spine	Flexion – slightly reduced due to pain Extension – full Side flexion and rotation – slightly reduced to left, full to right Tender C5/6 on the left
Upper limb neurology	No sensory or motor loss Reflexes intact

Approach to be taken

A. Data gathering, examination and clinical assessment skills

1. *Define the clinical problem: clarify why the patient has presented today*
The doctor:
- reads the patient information provided prior to the consultation – notes the past history of lower limb fractures and raised BMI and BP
- asks open questions to explore and clarify:
  - how Mr AB's neck pain affects him at home and at work
  - Mr AB's feelings about his weight and dieting
  - Mr AB's home circumstances
- empathises with Mr AB over work and home situations
- asks closed questions to exclude 'red flag' symptoms regarding his neck, metabolic causes for his obesity, and to assess his CVD risk
- discovers AB's feelings about medication and his fear that arthritis is hereditary
- uses internal summaries for each area to check that he has obtained the correct information

2. *Performs an appropriate physical or mental examination*
- In this case, an examination is appropriate and should include:
  - posture – cervical spine movements and quick upper limb neurology check for sensation; the patient reports no neurological symptoms, so a detailed neurological examination is not necessary
  - cardiovascular – BP and BMI at minimum; calculate CVD risk
- There is probably insufficient time to consider endocrine problems – hypothyroidism, Cushing's, diabetes, etc. These could be deferred to a follow-up appointment as he feels well.
- Explain the purpose of examination in appropriate language.
- The examination addresses the patient's ideas that his work is causing his pain and his concerns that he is developing neck arthritis.

B. Clinical management skills

3. *Make an appropriate working diagnosis*
The doctor:
- integrates information from the past and occupational histories, the pattern of pain, and the examination findings, to make a working diagnosis of postural neck pain
- identifies that Mr AB has an increased CVD risk due to obesity, BP, lack of exercise, and family history

4. Explain the problem to the patient using appropriate language
The doctor:
- addresses Mr AB's agenda:
  - neck pain is probably due to the work-station set-up
  - Mr AB's weight and lifestyle are increasing his risk of CVD
- provides information on posture and workplace set-up, CVD, and losing weight
- explains the need to monitor Mr AB's BP and weight, and for him to modify his lifestyle
- uses 'chunking and checking' to ensure accuracy of data collection and to check Mr AB's understanding at various stages throughout the consultation

5. Provide holistic care and use resources effectively
The doctor:
- practises evidence-based medicine – NICE obesity guidelines
- discusses the role of the occupational nurse to assess his workplace
- involves other members of the PHCT, such as the Practice Nurse, to give dietary advice and monitor Mr AB's weight and BP
- understands socioeconomic/cultural background – job losses and having to look after his arthritic mother
- demonstrates to Mr AB that the management of his problems share common features such as losing weight and increasing physical activity

6. Prescribe appropriately
The doctor:
- is aware of national and local guidelines (NICE guidelines on obesity and hypertension), and so dietary advice but not medication is indicated here
- reassures Mr AB that the use of intermittent ibuprofen and paracetamol is appropriate to help when pain interferes with work. The doctor should check that there are no contraindications to NSAID use such as indigestion and asthma.
- makes appropriate referral to physiotherapy for advice on self-management
- arranges further checks of BP and weight
- arranges dietary advice
- provides a letter for Mr AB's occupational nurse

7. Specify the conditions and interval for follow-up
The doctor:
- signposts Mr AB to information on posture and exercise, and weight management and healthy eating
- offers a follow-up appointment to check progress at work
- offers a follow-up appointment with the Practice Nurse to monitor weight and BP
- confirms understanding

C. Interpersonal skills: know and treat this patient

8. *Achieve rapport*

   The doctor:
   - listens attentively to Mr AB's concerns about his work and home situations
   - recognises verbal and non-verbal cues – Mr AB is reluctant to make a fuss at work as he is concerned about his job security
   - places problem in psychosocial context – how it may affect his ability to look after his mother
   - understands his request for physiotherapy and for a letter to his employers
   - discovers patient's health beliefs, e.g. that his workplace is contributing to his symptoms
   - addresses the patient's specific concerns and expectations

9. *Give the patient the opportunity to be involved in significant management decisions*

   The doctor:
   - encourages autonomy and opinions – provides patient with information and a letter to the occupational nurse to enable patient to tackle the cause of his neck pain
   - supports him in caring for his mother and explores whether additional help is required and would be acceptable to them

Debrief

This case could develop in several directions. The presenting complaint, neck pain, is relatively straightforward and the occupational cause should be identified readily. This should leave time to discuss Mr AB's weight problem and risks of CVD. However, there are other issues such as job insecurity and his mother's arthritis and increasing dependence on him that could deflect the doctor from completing the consultation in the available time.

Discuss how the doctor could, if needed, improve his performance. In particular, assess whether the doctor:
- identified that the neck pain was likely to be an occupational problem
- explored a range of management options with Mr AB – self-management exercises, posture advice, occupational nurse referral to name a few
- took the opportunity to talk about Mr AB's weight problem and the long-term effects of this on his health
- explored Mr AB's health beliefs and motivated him to lose weight and become more active
- arranged suitable investigation (work station assessment) and review

Revising data gathering

What questions could the doctor ask to discover the patient's ideas, concerns, expectations and health beliefs?
- Ideas: "*What do you think may have caused the neck pain?*".
- Concerns: "*Are you concerned about your weight?*".
- Expectations: "*It seems that your work may be causing your neck pain, shall we talk about how you might be able to improve things there?*".
- Health beliefs:
  - "*Your father died of a heart attack at quite a young age, are you worried that this might affect you?*"
  - "*You seem reluctant to take tablets for the neck pain, but if the pain is bad and affecting you, they can be useful, as correcting your posture and workplace may take some time to help things.*".

Once the doctor has gathered sufficient information, how could he summarise the problem for the patient?
- "*We have discussed a lot of issues today, and I would like to summarise back to you in case I've left out anything important or got anything wrong*".
- "*Your neck pain is most likely to be caused by your new work place; we have talked about how you might improve this at work and also about improving your posture. We have agreed that if things get worse, physiotherapy may ease the symptoms, but will not treat the cause, which you seem keen to tackle first*".
- "*We have discussed your risk of developing CVD given your family history, your increasing weight and BP. We have agreed to arrange some diet advice and support to lose weight and explore ways you can increase your physical activity*".

Relevant literature

NICE (2014), *Obesity: identification, assessment and management:* <u>tinyurl.com/CS3e-Lc2a</u> (*takes you to* <u>www.nice.org.uk/guidance/cg189/chapter/1-recommendations</u>)

National Obesity Forum, Guidelines on the management of adult obesity and overweight in primary care:
<u>www.nationalobesityforum.org.uk</u>

Background information

- Use body mass index (BMI) as a practical estimate of adiposity in adults (supplement with waist circumference for BMI <35).
- Interpret BMI with caution, particularly in highly muscular adults or those of Asian origin.
- Investigate comorbidities and other factors to an appropriate level, depending on the person, timing of assessment, degree of overweight or obesity, and previous assessments.
- In adults, consider referral to tier 3 specialist weight management services if the underlying cause needs to be assessed, their needs cannot be managed adequately in tier 2 with lifestyle interventions alone (such as those with learning disabilities), conventional treatment is unsuccessful, or drug treatment is being considered in those with BMI >50. People should have relevant information on realistic targets for weight loss (5–10% of original weight).
- To prevent obesity, most people may need to do 45–60 minutes of moderate intensity activity a day, particularly if they do not reduce their energy intake. Advise people who have been obese and have lost weight that they may need to do 60–90 minutes of activity a day to avoid regaining weight.
- Consider drug treatment (for adults) only after dietary, exercise, and behavioural approaches have been started and evaluated, and a target weight loss has not been reached or a plateau has been reached.
- Drug treatment is generally not recommended for children under 12 years unless severe comorbidities are present.
- Bariatric surgery is a treatment option if BMI is 40 or more (or 35–40 in the presence of comorbidities such as type 2 diabetes or high blood pressure), all appropriate non-surgical measures have been tried but the person does not achieve or maintain weight loss, the person is already being treated or will be treated in a tier 3 specialist weight management service, the person is fit for anaesthesia and surgery, and the person commits to the need for long-term follow-up.
- Bariatric surgery is the option of choice (instead of lifestyle interventions or drug treatment) for adults with a BMI of >50 when other interventions have not been effective.

Long case 3 – Childhood eczema

Brief to the doctor

Mrs CC is a 36 year old woman who presents (without her son) asking for a repeat prescription for his eczema. She hands you a list of his medication.

Patient summary

Name	Darius C
Date of birth (Age)	2
Social and Family History	Only child, parents aged 36 and 33
Past medical history	Treated for an 'eczema flare' 4 weeks ago with antibiotics and eumovate Seen in dermatology OPD 9 months ago – atopic eczema
Repeat medication	Doublebase thrice daily Aveeno at night Hydrocortisone as required or once daily for 7 days Oilatum Plus – use daily in bath

Tasks for the doctor

In this case, the tasks are to:
- clarify Mrs CC's concerns regarding her son's treatments
- review Darius' treatments, particularly efficacy and compliance
- prescribe appropriately

Brief to the patient – more about the patient

1. Profile:

- Mrs CC is a 36 year old woman who has returned to work (part-time) as an administrator
- married with 1 child, Darius, who has had eczema since infancy
- Mrs CC is worried about the severity of her son's eczema

2. She is seeing the doctor today because:

- she requires a repeat prescription of his medication
- she needs a set of emollients for nursery
- she recently attended a dinner party where one of the other guests, a health visitor, spoke to her about a new treatment, an 'anti-cancer' cream for eczema and she wants to talk to you about this
- she has not changed Darius' diet – should she?
- her mother-in-law is keen on taking Darius to see a local homeopath
- when asked about her application of the creams, she talks about applying the treatments conscientiously; she is concerned about nursery – they have only used one tube in three weeks and she uses a tube every week

3. Additional information:

- if the doctor discusses tacrolimus or pimecrolimus with her, she says she would like to read up about this before making a decision; she expects the doctor to signpost her to suitable information
- if Mrs CC feels comfortable with you, she volunteers her opinion on homeopathy – 'it is a load of drivel', however she would like your opinion; she also reveals her concern about her mother-in-law's interference, which she perceives as indirect criticism of her child raising

Approach to be taken

A. Data gathering, examination and clinical assessment skills

1. *Define the clinical problem: clarify why the patient has presented today*
   The doctor:
   - reads the patient information provided prior to the consultation
   - asks open questions to explore how Darius is getting on with his treatment, the bathing and 'creaming' routine, his recovery from his recent flare, and what she thought helped him to improve
   - empathises with her comments about how long the routine takes; this 'connection' with Mrs CC allows her to air her concerns regarding her suspicions that the nursery is not applying the emollients as diligently as she does at home
   - asks closed questions to clarify details about the current appearance of the skin and which parts of the body are affected
   - asks about current infection (weeping, pustules, malaise), facial eczema, sleep disturbance and nursery attendance, i.e. the doctor excludes red flags signalling the need for review or referral
   - discovers Mrs CC's idea that homeopathy is 'drivel', her concern about nursery, her expectation for further information about tacrolimus / pimecrolimus and her health belief that diet may be linked to eczema

2. *Performs an appropriate physical or mental examination*
   - In this case, an examination is not required.

B. Clinical management skills

3. *Make an appropriate working diagnosis*
   - The doctor, based on the history, makes a working diagnosis of childhood atopic eczema; Mrs CC tells you that the dermatologists agreed with this diagnosis and initiated the current treatment regime.

4. *Explain the problem to the patient using appropriate language*
   The doctor:
   - having quickly established that Mrs CC is sensible and diligent in her application of the creams, addresses her agenda
   - prescribes the medication and asks what she intends to do about nursery
   - provides some information on the effectiveness of complementary and alternative (CAM) treatments – very little of it has good trial evidence and some may be harmful, for example, some Chinese herbal medicines for eczema have been found to contain dexamethasone
   - explains that the health visitor may have been talking about tacrolimus or pimecrolimus; these immune suppressors may be useful for patients with moderate-to-severe disease, however, there is a theoretical increased risk

of developing skin cancer; they should be initiated by dermatologists or GPs with a special interest in dermatology, so it may be useful to discuss at the next OPD appointment

- advises Mrs CC that most children with atopic eczema do not have food allergy, and that exclusion diets rarely help. The importance of having a healthy balanced diet for growth and well-being is discussed.

5. *Provide holistic care and use resources effectively*
The doctor:
- practises evidence-based medicine
- is informed by national or local guidelines
- if Mrs CC is not overly concerned about the side-effects of steroid creams, then the doctor should not waste time addressing this issue – time is better spent addressing her concerns about diet and homeopathy

6. *Prescribe appropriately*
The doctor:
- is aware of national and local guidelines – tinyurl.com/CS3e-Lc3a (*takes you to* www.nice.org.uk/guidance/...) and tinyurl.com/CS3e-Lc3b (*takes you to* www.pcds.org.uk/.../pcdsbad-eczema.pdf)
- checks the patient's understanding of the medication and the amounts of medication required

7. *Specify the conditions and interval for follow-up*
The doctor:
- signposts Mrs CC to information on tacrolimus or pimecrolimus – tinyurl.com/CS3e-Lc3c (*takes you to* www.nice.org.uk/...topical-calcineurin-inhibitors)
- offers a follow-up appointment to discuss any issues arising from her reading; it would be useful to review Darius 'in the flesh' at this appointment to assess whether he meets criteria for initiation of these drugs

C. Interpersonal skills: know and treat this patient

8. *Achieve rapport*
The doctor:
- listens attentively to Mrs CC's concerns about nursery and her mother-in-law
- understands her request for information on alternative treatments
- displays empathy to the time-consuming routine and chronicity of the illness
- is non-judgemental about the patient's ideas on homeopathy and 'anti-cancer' creams
- addresses the patient's specific concerns and expectations

9. *Give the patient the opportunity to be involved in significant management decisions*
The doctor:
- encourages autonomy and opinions – provides her with information so she feels able to tackle treatment issues with nursery and her mother-in-law
- supports and congratulates her in caring for her son

Debrief

Discuss how the doctor could, if needed, improve his performance. In particular, assess whether the doctor:
- established rapport? If so, how?
- addressed Mrs CC's specific concerns? If so, how?
- discussed the evidence base for immune suppressors, exclusion diets and CAM?
- explained the risks and benefits of treatments in simple language?

If the consultation over-ran, did the doctor:
- repeat certain questions when taking the history?
- repeat some explanations?
- address issues the patient was not concerned about?

Revising data gathering

- What questions could the doctor ask to discover the patient's ideas, concerns, expectations and health beliefs?
- Ideas: *"I understand that your mother-in-law is keen on homeopathy. What is your view?"*
- Concerns: *"I agree that if applied as prescribed, nursery should have run out of cream much sooner. Are you concerned that they may not be applying the cream as directed?"*
- Expectations: *"It seems to me your recent discussion with the health visitor led to you to think about alternative treatments. I'll quickly outline the risks and benefits of these immune suppressor creams."*
- Health beliefs: *"You suspect that diet and eczema may be linked. Let's talk about this for a moment."*

Relevant literature

tinyurl.com/CS3e-Lc3b (*takes you to* www.pcds.org.uk/.../pcdsbad-eczema.pdf)

www.sign.ac.uk/pdf/sign125.pdf

tinyurl.com/CS3e-Lc3a (*takes you to* www.nice.org.uk/guidance/..)

Background information

- Teach patients and parents how to recognise flares of atopic eczema (increased dryness, itching, redness, swelling and general irritability).
- Treatment for flares of atopic eczema in children should be started as soon as signs and symptoms appear and continued for approximately 48 hours after symptoms subside.
- Offer children with atopic eczema a choice of unperfumed emollients to use every day for moisturising, washing and bathing. Leave-on emollients should be prescribed in large quantities (250–500 g weekly) and easily available to use at nursery, pre-school or school.
- Review repeat prescriptions at least once a year to ensure that therapy remains optimal.
- Use a mild potency steroid for the face and neck, except for short-term (3–5 days) use of moderate potency for severe flares.
- Use moderate or potent preparations for short periods only (7–14 days) for flares in vulnerable sites such as axillae and groin.
- A different topical corticosteroid of the same potency should be considered as an alternative to stepping up treatment if tachyphylaxis to a topical corticosteroid is suspected in children with atopic eczema.
- It is recommended that treatment with tacrolimus (licensed in patients under age 2) or pimecrolimus (age 2–16) be initiated only by physicians (including general practitioners) with a special interest and experience in dermatology, and only after careful discussion with the patient about the potential risks and benefits of all appropriate second-line treatment options.

Long case 4 – Tennis elbow

Brief to the doctor

Mrs CD is a 28 year old lady who presents with a right tennis elbow.

Patient summary

Name	CD
Date of birth (Age)	28
Social and family history	Married No children No recorded FH of CVD, DM
Past medical history	Seen 4 months ago: *"Repeat COCP. No problems."* Seen 3 months ago: *"Persistent headaches – few weeks. Nil specific. Not unwell. Denies any worries. Diagnosis ?cause. Take OTC analgesia if reqd. Suggest watch and wait."* Seen 1 month ago: *"Pain Rt shoulder/neck – 2 weeks. No cause identified. Full range of mvmt neck and shoulder. Declined analgesia. Offered physio but declined this as well."*
Current medication	COCP

Investigations	
BP	3 months ago
	132/86
HR	84
	2 years ago – normal cervical smear
Smokes	<10/day

Tasks for the doctor

In this case, the tasks are to:
- assess the severity of Mrs CD's tennis elbow and agree a management plan
- respond to cues about her marriage and sensitively explore her satisfaction with her marriage and how she might try to improve the situation

Brief to the patient – more about the patient

1. Profile:

- Mrs CD is a 28 year old lady who is married to a leading local businessman who is 50 years old; they have a very comfortable lifestyle – large house, expensive cars and holidays
- she gave up her job as an art teacher when she married 4 years ago – she is frustrated that she is no longer working and gave up a profession
- she tries to occupy herself, but finds this difficult. She had to leave a local art group, which she really enjoyed, because her husband became very jealous that she was mixing with like-minded people, some of whom were her age and male. He has enrolled her in the tennis section at the golf club where he is a member and has bought her lessons there. He takes her to the club and plays golf with business acquaintances while she has lessons, then expects her to help entertain his guests over lunch.
- she feels she is used as a glamorous and vivacious 'trophy wife'
- she would like children, but her husband will not consider this as he feels children would distract him from work and prevent him enjoying his current lifestyle

2. She is seeing the doctor today because:

- her right elbow is sore after tennis; she thinks she can probably cope with it, but her husband has insisted she consult, in case it is something serious
- the elbow does not hurt at any other time. Her husband noticed it because she complained that her elbow hurt when driving him home after a business lunch. There has never been any swelling or loss of movement, nor any neurological symptoms. Her neck pain has gone.
- she does not expect or want any treatment. She would be very happy to be told to rest and avoid tennis for a while. She is not at all keen on medicines and prefers to use 'natural' remedies whenever possible.

3. Additional information:

- if the doctor asks specifically:
  - she feels very unhappy with her life and her marriage in particular – she regrets getting married and feels trapped
  - if pressed, she would accept that her presentations with persistent headaches, sore neck/shoulder and elbow pain are reflections of her unhappiness
- she would like the opportunity to talk about how she feels, but only after the doctor has given her enough time and information to enable her to reassure her husband that her elbow pain has been taken seriously. She will not raise

the subject, but will talk freely if the doctor raises the issue. She hopes that by dropping cues that she feels pressured into playing, and that she is not that bothered if told to rest completely, the doctor will suspect there is another matter she wishes to raise. However, if he asks her "*Is there anything else you want to talk about?*" without putting this into context, she will answer "*no*". She feels that the last doctor that saw her realised there was something else going on, but attempted to 'fob her off' by offering her physiotherapy.

- if asked:
  - she watches her weight very carefully as her husband criticises her if she gains any
  - she has trouble getting to sleep and wakes several times every night
  - she gets tearful easily and tries to avoid talking or thinking about her life because doing so upsets her
  - she has briefly considered suicide but dismissed the idea instantly as she wants to enjoy life not get out of it
  - she feels her parents would be very unsupportive as they disapproved of her marrying someone older and she thinks their attitude would be 'told you so' which she thinks would not be helpful; she is an only child
  - she has no close friends currently; however, she occasionally contacts an old boyfriend who is always very sympathetic and supportive – she occasionally thinks she should have married him
- if the doctor examines her:

System	Findings
Neck	Full range of movement Posture normal
Shoulder	Full range of movement Normal scapulothoracic rhythm
Elbow	Flexion/extension – full and pain-free Pronation/supination – full and pain-free No effusion Very slight tenderness on deep palpation over the lateral epicondyle No pain on resisted wrist dorsiflexion
Forearm	No swelling or tenderness
Neuro	No altered sensation or weakness; reflexes intact Neural tension tests negative

Approach to be taken

A. Data gathering, examination and clinical assessment skills

1. *Define the clinical problem: clarify why the patient has presented today*
   The doctor:
   - reads the patient information provided prior to the consultation, identifying several recent consultations for 'minor' problems
   - asks open questions to explore the presenting reason for her attendance (husband's concern), to clarify her symptoms (minor) and to ascertain how they affect her (minimally)
   - asks closed questions to exclude the neck as a cause of her pain
   - listens attentively and responds to cues such as her feeling pressurised into playing tennis
   - explores whether there are other issues she wishes to discuss using open and closed questions, silence and reference to previous attendances

2. *Performs an appropriate physical or mental examination*
   - In this case, a targeted examination is required – the minimally acceptable examination would be to exclude restricted elbow joint movement (flexion, extension, pronation and supination) and localised swelling or tenderness
   - the examination should address the patient's (and her husband's) concerns
   - a 'gold standard' examination would include neck and shoulder movements and systematic examination of the upper limb

B. Clinical management skills

3. *Make an appropriate working diagnosis*
   The doctor:
   - integrates information from previous consultations, questions about her presenting complaint, cues and questions about her happiness
   - identifies and explores, by using a patient-centred approach, the real reason for the patient's attendance
   - makes a working diagnosis of mild tennis elbow and underlying marital unhappiness

4. *Explain the problem to the patient using appropriate language*
   The doctor:
   - having quickly established that this was a case of mild tennis elbow, gives appropriate management advice – rest from tennis
   - agrees with the patient that medication and referral for physiotherapy are not appropriate
   - provides some information on the effectiveness of complementary and alternative (CAM) treatments – acupuncture/dry needling, and exercises and self-management techniques may help. See examples of

a rehabilitation and graduated loading programme at www.bmj.com/
content/342/bmj.d2687

5. *Provide holistic care and use resources effectively*
The doctor:
- does not make an unnecessary physiotherapy referral or prescribe
  analgesia
- by exploring the socioeconomic/cultural background, is likely to discover
  the real reason for the attendance

6. *Prescribe appropriately*
The doctor:
- agrees not to prescribe any medication – analgesics and non-steroidal
  anti-inflammatory drugs can be used to help patients cope with the pain
  of tennis elbow, which is hopefully temporary; these drugs do not improve
  the long-term outcome of the condition
- explores a range of management strategies to deal with her unhappiness –
  how she might raise her frustration at no longer working and having to be a
  'trophy wife' with her husband

7. *Specify the conditions and interval for follow-up*
The doctor:
- offers a follow-up to explore her feelings about her marriage

C. Interpersonal skills: know and treat this patient

8. *Achieve rapport*
The doctor:
- listens attentively to Mrs CD's explanations of her symptoms
- explores and clarifies her symptoms and feelings
- recognises verbal and non-verbal cues – not being concerned about having
  to rest from tennis
- sensitively explores Mrs CD's unhappiness with her marriage and
  frustration with her lifestyle
- places the problem in psychosocial context – her husband pressurising her
  to play tennis
- discovers the patient's health beliefs and understands her reluctance to
  have medication

9. *Give the patient the opportunity to be involved in significant management decisions*
The doctor:
- actively confirms patient's understanding of the problem, i.e. that her
  tennis elbow is mild and requires rest from the aggravating activity
- supports and empathises with her marital unhappiness
- explores various strategies for improving her lifestyle and hence happiness

Debrief

The presenting symptom, tennis elbow, is minor and the real issue in this consultation is picking up the patient's cues about her marriage and then exploring this issue.

Discuss how the doctor could, if needed, improve his performance. In particular, assess how the doctor:

- established rapport with Mrs CD
- identified the underlying issue
- explored strategies Mrs CD might employ to raise or address her unhappiness

Revising data gathering

What questions could the doctor ask to discover the patient's ideas, concerns, expectations and health beliefs?

- Ideas: *"On a scale of 0–5, with 5 being catastrophic, how serious do you think the problem with your elbow is?"*
- Concerns: *"You said that your husband has made you come today, why do you think he has done that?"*
- Expectations: *"It seems to me that the last few times you have come here you have had problems that you didn't want any treatment for. Sometimes that happens when people are worried about something else and so I wonder if there is another problem, perhaps a personal one, that you would like to discuss?"*
- Health beliefs: *"I see you were not keen on painkillers before, is that because you don't like taking medicines?"*

Once the doctor has gathered sufficient information, how could he summarise the problem for the patient?

- *"Your elbow pain does not seem to interfere with you that much and my examination is pretty normal"*

If the consultation over-ran, did the doctor:

- allow the patient to repeat herself or not offer useful information?
- not understand why the patient had attended?
- not pick up the patient's cues?
- find it difficult discussing personal issues and feelings with the patient?
- spend too much time data gathering and not enough time listening?
- fail to organise and structure the consultation appropriately?

Relevant literature

Bisset L, Paungmail A, Vicenzino B, *et al.* (2005) A systematic review and meta-analysis of clinical trials on physical interventions for lateral epicondylalagia. *Br J Sports Med,* **39**: 411–422.

YouTube (www.youtube.com/watch?v=yRkDTTn1FvA) – video discussing eccentric exercises for tennis elbow.

tinyurl.com/CS3e-Lc4a (*takes you to* www.arthritisresearchuk.org/...tennis-elbow-exercises.aspx) – exercises to manage tennis elbow.

Background information

- A diagnosis of tennis elbow is often made on the basis of clinical assessment. Radiography and ultrasound are not usually needed.
- The initial aim of management is to reduce tendon load; educate patients about the pathology and activities that would overload the tendon. Advise patients to reduce their lifting activities and limit the amount of time spent using a computer.
- As the pain gradually subsides because of the load reduction, formal eccentric exercises can be started, increasing in intensity gradually as guided by pain, although patients should not be discouraged from performing exercises with a low degree of pain (<5 out of 10 pain on subjective assessment). Simultaneously, scapular and shoulder stability exercises are also recommended.
- Inform patients about the importance of maintaining the rehabilitation programme, even after returning to full work duties. If the recovery halts or the pain worsens, other treatments are available, such as platelet-rich plasma injections and nitrate patches.

Long case 5 – Ankle injury

Brief to the doctor

Mr TP is a 22 year old man who presents with a sore ankle (right). He walks into your surgery on crutches. He is due to leave for Ghana in 5 weeks as part of a VSO team.

Patient summary

Name	TP
Date of birth (Age)	22
Social and Family History	Unmarried
Past medical history	Tonsillitis 3 years ago Insomnia 6 years ago
Current medication	None
Blood tests	Tests were done 4 months ago (VSO medical)
BMI	27
BP	128/68

Tasks for the doctor

In this case, the tasks are to:
- assess how the ankle injury impacts on his life
- provide him with information about healing times
- help him to reach a decision about physiotherapy and his fitness to undertake volunteer work in a remote area

Brief to the patient – more about the patient

1. Profile:

- Mr TP is a 22 year old man
- unmarried and not currently in a relationship
- works with his father in the building trade undertaking barn conversions and building renovations
- due to start a 3-month VSO placement in Ghana in 5 weeks
- injured his ankle during a football game with his mates 7 days ago; attended A&E where an X-ray ruled out an ankle fracture – he was told to take analgesia and to see his GP for further treatment
- in the week since the injury, he has mobilised well on crutches, is now weight-bearing on the ankle and takes one 400 mg ibuprofen thrice daily

2. He is seeing the doctor today because:

- the A&E doctor told him he didn't have a fracture but didn't give any advice about mobilizing or running
- the box of tablets he was given says he should take one tablet three times a day after meals – for how long should he continue with the tablets?
- he has tried putting weight through the ankle and has walked from his bed to the toilet without crutches – although it was painful (5/10), it was bearable
- what should he do about crutches; when can he start running again; does he need physiotherapy?
- he would like to know if his ankle will be healed within 5 weeks; he is worried about letting his VSO team members down if he needs extra help or if he cannot carry out certain physical tasks such as helping to build a water pipe; also, in Ghana, he will be living in a remote rural area some distance from medical care
- when he contacted VSO for advice, they advised him to consult his GP first
- he does not have private health insurance; if you advise him to pay to see a physiotherapist, he is happy to do so, especially if you think physiotherapy can get his ankle strong again for his Ghana trip
- if the doctor offers him a 'wait and see' policy, he wants to know what he should tell VSO
- if the doctor offers him an NHS physiotherapy referral, he wants to know the likelihood of being seen within 5 weeks
- by the way, he has season tickets to the local football club (worth approximately £550); his parents don't go to games, so would the doctor like the tickets? He is grateful to the practice for organising his VSO medical at short notice and for waiving their fee.

Approach to be taken

A. Data gathering, examination and clinical assessment skills

1. *Define the clinical problem: clarify why the patient has presented today*
   The doctor:
   - notes, from the medical record, that Mr TP had a VSO medical 4 months ago
   - detects a non-verbal cue – Mr TP walks in on crutches; on questioning the reason for the crutches, the doctor obtains a history of the ankle injury and the hospital treatment
   - asks open questions to explore what specifically about the ankle injury brings him to the surgery today, i.e. the doctor explores his expectations and concerns
   - asks focused and closed questions to clarify details of the pain, analgesia, and ability to mobilize
   - elicits how the problem affects Mr TP and discovers his concerns about being fit to travel to Ghana in 5 weeks as part of a VSO team
   - explores his health beliefs that physiotherapy would lead to quicker healing
   - summarises the problem: as regards your ankle sprain, you are consulting today for advice on painkillers, when to restart running, and whether you should go to Ghana in 5 weeks – have I understood you correctly?

2. *Perform an appropriate physical or mental examination*
   - An examination of the ankle is unlikely to be needed given the history of improvements (in pain and mobility) and the fact that the patient does not have specific concerns warranting physical reassessment.

B. Clinical management skills

3. *Make an appropriate working diagnosis*
   The doctor:
   - recognises from the history and examination that the patient is describing a typical grade 2 ankle sprain
   - recognises that the ankle injury is healing as it should be (i.e. following the expected pattern of illness); non-operative treatment with early functional rehabilitation is the treatment of choice

4. *Explain the problem to the patient using appropriate language*
   The doctor:
   - is patient-centred – uses the patient's ideas on mobilizing (without crutches) as pain allows, reducing NSAIDs and perhaps changing to topical NSAIDs or analgesics, and starting rehabilitation of the ankle (explaining that running may not be the best way to achieve ankle strength and stability – www.bmj.com/content/339/bmj.b2901)

- uses the patient's beliefs regarding physiotherapy – explains that initial physiotherapy treatment with ultrasound or infrared attempts to reduce swelling and pain, and that later rehabilitation teaches stretching and strengthening exercises to prevent re-injury
- provides information on healing times: grade 2 sprains – people usually start walking on the ankle after 2 days of rest; the swelling goes down after 7–10 days; people in physically demanding jobs may take a few weeks to return to work and people may not be able to take part in sport for a few months
- addresses the patient's concerns and expectations – explores the risks and benefits of postponing the VSO trip until the ankle has regained full strength (this may take a few months) versus going to Ghana where walking on uneven ground may put an incompletely healed ankle at risk of re-injury

5. *Provide holistic care and use resources effectively*
   The doctor:
   - may, after discussion with the patient, refer to physiotherapy (NHS or private based on his preference)
   - practises evidence-based medicine
   - is informed by national or local guidelines – www.bmj.com/content/339/bmj.b2901

6. *Prescribe appropriately*
   The doctor:
   - is aware of national and local guidelines
   - chooses cost-effective medication (paracetamol rather than codeine; ibuprofen rather than alternative NSAIDs)
   - checks the patient's understanding of the medication and warns the patient about potential side effects

7. *Specify the conditions and interval for follow-up*
   - The doctor outlines expected healing times and advises the patient to return for re-assessment if he does not heal as predicted

C. Interpersonal skills: know and treat this patient

8. *Achieve rapport*
   The doctor:
   - understands how important the VSO trip is to him and displays empathy with his bad luck
   - addresses the patient's specific concerns (about rehabilitation) and his expectations regarding VSO
   - thanks the patient for his offer of the football tickets, which raises an ethical issue: does the offer affect the doctor's decision-making in any way; how does the doctor politely refuse the gift; if the gift is accepted, does the

doctor explain to Mr TP the new stipulation in the GP contract that GPs keep a register of gifts with a value over £100?

9. *Give the patient the opportunity to be involved in significant management decisions*
The doctor:
- shares his thoughts on healing times, the value of rehabilitation and involves the patient in decisions
- encourages autonomy and opinions – asks Mr TP questions that allow him to evaluate the benefits and risks of going to Ghana in 5 weeks, thus facilitating his decision-making

Debrief

Discuss how the doctor could, if needed, improve his performance. In particular, assess whether the doctor:

- understood the reason for the patient's attendance today or whether he made assumptions regarding the patient's agenda? If so, what questions or explanations did the doctor use that led him down this incorrect track?
- asked questions that facilitated Mr TP's decision-making or did the doctor make decisions for him?
- deal with the gift ethically and sensitively?

If the consultation over-ran:

- did the doctor repeat his questions or explanations?
- perform any unnecessary examinations?
- get embarrassed or flummoxed by the gift?

Revising data gathering

What questions could the doctor ask to discover the patient's ideas, concerns, expectations and health beliefs?

- Ideas: *"I understand that you want your ankle to heal as fast as possible. Did you have any ideas on how we could achieve this?"*
- Concerns: *"What is your ankle injury preventing you from doing, at work or socially? Is there anything in particular about your fitness that concerns you?"*
- Expectations: *"When you came into surgery today, what is it that you hoped I would do for you?"*
- Health beliefs: *"Am I right in thinking that you believe the ankle will heal faster with physiotherapy? Let's talk about what improves ankle healing in the short and long term."*

List to the podcast from 2 min 20 to 6 min 30 to hear the discussion on ICE – tinyurl.com/CS3e-Lc5a (*takes you to* https://soundcloud.com/bmjpodcasts/...)

Relevant literature

http://bjsm.bmj.com/content/36/2/83.full
www.bmj.com/content/339/bmj.b2901

Background information

Ankle sprains can be classified into three levels of severity:
- Grade I is stretching with minor tear of the ligament and with no signs of laxity;
- Grade II is a partial tear; and
- Grade III is a complete tear of the ligament.

All but the most severe can be placed in a dynamic splinting device such as the Aircastand, tubular dressings, the Bledsoe boot (complex immobilisation boot), Aircast, and below knee cylinder cast for patients with severe ankle sprains. Those treated by plaster immobilisation with a below knee cast or either of the dynamic immobilisation devices had more rapid healing of their ankle sprains at three months than did those treated with a tubular bandage, and the costs of the cast or Aircast were minimally higher than the plaster cast. Nine months after injury, all groups had equal functional outcomes.

With more serious injury, physical therapy may be helpful.

Serious injuries that should not be missed are complete disruption of the fibulotalar or deltoid ligaments, mortise, or interosseous ligament, which could require surgical repair to restore a functional and stable ankle. Suspect these if patients continue to have severe pain after a few days of rest and if they have laxity or severe pain when the ligaments are under stress. Ligamentous laxity is tested for with the "drawer test", which looks for appreciable movement of the forefoot relative to the ankle or severe pain when the ligaments are stressed, leading to suspicion of complete ligamentous disruption.

Long case 6 – MRI result – back pain

Brief to the doctor

Mr EF, age 42, wishes to discuss the treatment options for his back following a recent MRI scan organised by the hospital orthopaedic department. He has previously been seeing one of your partners who is now on maternity leave.

Patient summary

Name	EF
Date of birth (Age)	42
Past medical history	1 year ago – GP notes: *"LBP with Rt L5 pain and paraesthesia – 3 months. Private physio and osteopath have not helped. Ibuprofen and Co-codamol 30/500 (prescribed by dental colleague) not helped. V stiff L spine. SLR 30 on Rt, 90 on Lt. Absent Ankle Jerk. Letter from physio suggesting referral. Refer Orthopaedics"*
	9 months ago – Letter from Specialist Physio Clinic: *"5 months LBP with L5 sciatica. No red flags. Has only had manipulative treatment in private sector, for outpatient physio."*
	7 months ago – GP notes: *"Hospital physio referred him for more physio – v unhappy. Getting worse. Interfering with ability to work, considering having to reduce workload, partners at work not happy with him. Wants to see orthopaedic consultant not physio. Letter to consultant requesting he review patient."*
	5 months ago – Consultant letter: *"Thank you for asking me to see Mr EF. I think the time has come to establish the cause of his back and leg pain and have arranged an MRI. I have warned him that there is likely to be a wait for this. I will see him when he has had the scan to discuss treatment options."*

2 weeks ago – MRI result: "*Reduced signal L4/5 and L5/S1 discs. There is a large Rt sided disc protrusion compressing the L5 root.*"

Current medication   Ibuprofen 400 mg 1 tab 3 or 4 times daily with food
Co-codamol 30/500 2 tabs 4 times daily as required

Tasks for the doctor

In this case, the tasks are to:

- explain the MRI result and treatment options to Mr EF
- explore his concerns about treatments and their long and short-term effects on his health and work (expectations)
- support and explore his disappointment with the quality of care he has received from the hospital

Brief to the patient – more about the patient

1. Profile:

- 42 year old partner in a local private dental practice and is married with 2 children aged 10 and 8 years
- he developed low back pain and right sciatica 15 months ago and initially saw an osteopath and then a physiotherapist privately, but did not respond to treatment. His physiotherapist advised that he needed a scan and possibly an operation. He therefore attended his GP and was referred to the orthopaedic department at the local hospital for an MRI.
- he was seen by a specialist physiotherapist at the hospital who was very critical of the treatment he had received from both the osteopath and from the physiotherapist. He was told there was no indication for an urgent scan and that he should attend the hospital outpatient physiotherapy department for 'proper' physiotherapy.
- he was very unhappy at not being seen by a consultant as he feels that it was discourteous to a fellow health practitioner; he was not happy with the clinic recommendations, but did not want to make a fuss and so complied with the recommendations
- attending physiotherapy outpatients was very disruptive to his practice as the department only offered appointments during the working day. He had already reduced his workload with his partners' agreement, but he sensed that they were getting disgruntled with his reduced presence and contribution to the practice.
- his symptoms did not respond to outpatient physiotherapy and so he saw his GP again and requested a consultant appointment. When he saw the consultant, he was immediately referred for an MRI scan.

2. He is seeing the doctor today because:

- he had the scan 2 weeks ago and would like to know the result
- he has an outpatient appointment in 6 weeks, and would like to discuss what treatments he is likely to be offered by the consultant
- he is concerned that he may never return to full working ability again, even after a back operation
- he wonders whether he would have got better and quicker treatment if he had been seen privately or if he had the MRI earlier
- if there is time, he would like to discuss making a complaint about the treatment he has received at the hospital, particularly the delay in getting the MRI

3. Additional information:

- if the doctor asks specifically:
  - he has constant back and leg pain and is kept awake by pain and so sleeps only fitfully

- he feels that his right leg is getting weak and the pins and needles are now constant. Coughing, sneezing and straining produce leg pain. He has no problems with bowel or bladder control and no perineal numbness. His weight is stable.
  - his pain is made worse by bending or twisting, which he has to do frequently at work
  - he is a keen runner but has not been able to run since his back pain started
  - the constant pain and lack of sleep are making him grumpy and short-tempered; while he manages to control this at work, if pressed, he has taken it out on his wife and children, but has never been violent.
- he is concerned that his business partners could ask him to leave the partnership or reduce his share of the profits due to his reduced workload. With 2 children at private school, he cannot afford to reduce his income.
- he believes that an operation is indicated and that if the hospital had listened to his GP and private physiotherapist, he could have had the operation by now and hence not be worrying about the effects on work, as well as sparing him and his family from the effects of his worsening symptoms
- he does not want an epidural and will refuse a referral to the Pain Clinic
- he trusts his GPs as they have always given him honest, sensible and unbiased advice
- he does not like to make a fuss and looks to his GP to be his advocate, but feels he should be treated as a priority due to the adverse effect of his problem on work and home
- he has some savings and has discussed with his wife whether to use these to fund an operation privately in order to get it done quickly
- if the doctor examines him:

System	Findings
General	Walks slowly and sits with difficulty Looks tired and drawn
Lumbar spine	Flattened lordosis Flexion-fingertips to top of patella Extension – nil Side flexion – reduced to the right more than to the left Tender palpation L4/5 and L5/S1 Spasm and tenderness of paraspinal muscles
Neurology	SLR 70 left with some cross pain, 20 right Slump test pos. on right Femoral stretch negative bilaterally Absent sensation L5 (right) Weak big toe extension and foot eversion (right) Absent ankle jerk (right)

Approach to be taken

A. Data gathering, examination and clinical assessment skills

1. Define the clinical problem: clarify why the patient has presented today
The doctor:
- reads the patient information provided prior to the consultation
- uses a well organised approach to gather information
- asks open questions to explore how Mr EF is getting on in terms of symptoms and how they are affecting his life – *"How is all this affecting you at work and home?"*
- asks closed questions to clarify details about level of pain, weakness and paraesthesia, and to exclude cauda equina symptoms
- discovers Mr EF's belief that an operation is required and that this should be done as soon as possible
- explores and clarifies the impact his symptoms are having on his home life

2. Performs an appropriate physical or mental examination
- In this case, an examination is required as Mr EF has indicated that his symptoms have worsened, in particular that he has developed weakness.
- A targeted examination should be made concentrating on lower limb neurology.

B. Clinical management skills

3. Make an appropriate working diagnosis
- The doctor integrates information from the history, scan result and examination, and makes a working diagnosis of L5 nerve root compression due to prolapsed lumbar intervertebral disc.

4. Explain the problem to the patient using appropriate language
The doctor:
- uses the patient's ideas and beliefs and explains the MRI result and indicates that the consultant is most likely to offer an operation – *"Do you know much about back operations?"*
- explains the natural history of prolapsed discs
- outlines the various options available while not pre-empting the consultant's opinion – operation, epidural, pain clinic
- provides some information on recovery times and functional outcomes from operations in order to address the patient's concerns
- reviews the effectiveness, or not, of Mr EF's current analgesia
- checks understanding – *"Does my explanation make sense? Is there anything else you would like to ask?"*

5. *Provide holistic care and use resources effectively*
The doctor:
- practises evidence-based medicine
- is informed by national or local guidelines
- understands and explores the socioeconomic background – effects on work and home life

6. *Prescribe appropriately*
The doctor:
- reviews Mr EF's current analgesia regimen and considers offering an alternative NSAID (+PPI), stronger opiates or neuropathic pain medication, such as TCA, duloxetine, gabapentin or pregabalin
- checks the patient's understanding of the medication and the amounts of medication required
- discovers whether Mr EF would like to elect for private treatment at this point in time or wait to see the outcome of the outpatient appointment
- decides whether to discuss the urgency of the case with the consultant based on the history and examination findings, but also in view of the patient's dissatisfaction with the treatment received thus far

7. *Specify the conditions and interval for follow-up*
- The doctor ensures Mr EF is aware of the 'red flag symptoms' – safety netting

C. Interpersonal skills: know and treat this patient

8. *Achieve rapport*
The doctor:
- listens attentively to Mr EF's description of his symptoms and their effect on work and home
- may use verbal and non-verbal cues to clarify the degree of Mr EF's disability: *"You seem to have difficulty moving around, is that causing you any problems?"*
- places problem in a psychosocial context – how it affects patient/family
- understands his request for information on recovery and success of treatments
- displays empathy – *"How are you coping?"*
- explores patient's health ideas, concerns and expectations
- is understanding but non-judgemental about the advice and opinion Mr EF was given in his initial hospital appointment; gives advice about making a complaint if Mr EF requests this
- supports Mr EF's efforts to continue working and remain active

9. *Give the patient the opportunity to be involved in significant management decisions*
The doctor:
- actively confirms the patient's understanding of the problem
- shares thoughts/involves patient in deciding how to progress management: *"There are a number of options here… Which of these do you prefer?"*

Debrief

Discuss how the doctor could, if needed, improve his performance. In particular, assess whether the doctor:
- achieved rapport
- dealt with Mr EF's unhappiness with aspects of his treatment by the hospital
- addressed Mr EF's concerns about the impact on his ability to work both in the short and the long term

If the consultation over-ran, did the doctor:
- manage the time available appropriately and in a structured and organised way?
- concentrate on addressing the issues Mr EF was most concerned about (impact on work and family life) or get bogged-down dealing with some aspects of the case (dissatisfaction with the hopsital)?

Revising data gathering

What questions could the doctor ask to discover the patient's ideas, concerns, expectations and health beliefs?
- Ideas: *"Now the scan has confirmed the clinical diagnosis of a disc prolapse, what treatment do you think the consultant is likely to recommend?"*.
- Concerns: *"You have told me that you feel under pressure from your partners because you have had to reduce your workload; how do you think they are going to feel if you have to have an operation?"*.
- Expectations: *"It seems to me that you believe you need an operation, would you like me to outline the basic options available to you?"*.
- Health beliefs: *"You seem concerned that your symptoms may not recover after an operation, would you like to discuss the success rates of operations with myself or the consultant?"*.

Relevant literature

Carragee EJ. (2005) The surgical treatment of disc degeneration: is the race not to be too swift? *Spine,* **5:** 587–588.

Gibson JN, Waddell G. (2007) Surgical interventions for lumbar disc prolapse. *Cochrane Database Syst Rev,* **1:** CD001350.

Koes BW, van Tulder MW, Peul WC. (2007) Diagnosis and treatment of sciatica. *BMJ,* **334:** 1313–1317.

Background information

Deyo RA *et al.* (2015) Opiates for low back pain. *BMJ*, **350**: g6380.

- Opioids seem to have short- (not long-) term analgesic efficacy for chronic back pain, but benefits for function are less clear.
- The magnitude of pain relief across chronic non-cancer pain conditions is about 30%, so you should expect 70% of your LBP patients on opiates not to have much relief, and you should therefore be discontinuing your prescription.
- The long-term effectiveness and safety of opioids are unknown. Loss of long-term efficacy could result from drug tolerance and emergence of hyperalgesia (increased sensitivity to pain, resulting perhaps from nerve damage).
- Complications of opioid use include addiction and overdose-related mortality.
- Common short-term side-effects are constipation, nausea, sedation and increased risk of falls and fractures.
- Longer-term side-effects may include depression and sexual dysfunction.
- Screening for high risk patients, treatment agreements and urine testing have not reduced overall rates of opioid prescribing, misuse or overdose.
- Newer strategies for reducing risks include more selective prescription of opioids and lower doses; use of prescription monitoring programmes; avoidance of co-prescription with sedative hypnotics.
- Newer strategies for reducing risk.

Long case 7 - Foot pain

Brief to the doctor

Mr SF is a 37 year old man who presents with a 4-day history of worsening foot pain (right). He requests analgesia. He had blood tests done 5 months ago and was advised to make lifestyle changes.

Patient summary

Name	SF
Date of birth (Age)	37
Social and Family History	Married, two children
	Dad fatal MI aged 69
Past medical history	Hypercholesterolaemia (5 months ago)
	Morton's neuroma 2nd left toe (1 year ago)
	Gout (2 years ago)
Current medication	None
Blood tests	Tests were done 5 months ago
Plasma fasting glucose	5.8 mmol/l (3.65–5.5)
Fasting cholesterol	7.2 mmol/l
Fasting HDL cholesterol	0.8 mmol/l (0.8–1.8)
Total cholesterol:HDL	9
TSH	1.89 (0.35–5.5)
Alkaline phosphatase	156 IU/l (95–280)
Total bilirubin	14 µmol/l (3–17)
Albumin	46 g/l (35–50)
Creatinine level	99 µmol/l (70–150)
BMI	34
BP	141/86
Framingham	12%
Plasma urate (2 years ago)	467 (210–480)

Tasks for the doctor

In this case, the tasks are to:
- advise Mr SF on analgesia and prescribe appropriately
- talk to Mr SF about his lifestyle changes
- arrange suitable follow-up

Brief to the patient - more about the patient

1. Profile:

- Mr SF is a 37 year old man
- married with 2 young children
- he works as an administrator for a logistics company, mainly office-based
- his dad died 6 months ago of a fatal MI; this prompted him to see his GP for a health check – his cholesterol was high
- he was told to reduce his cholesterol by changing his diet, taking more exercise and losing weight; he found dieting difficult; hence 2 weeks ago, he started a Slighter Lite programme of pre-prepared meals
- he had severe foot pain 2 years ago; he was told it was gout, but the follow-up blood test did not show a raised plasma urate so he is confused about the original diagnosis

2. He is seeing the doctor today because:

- he has severe pain in his right foot – he started taking ibuprofen 400 mg thrice daily because he suspected gout, but the foot remains painful; he wants stronger analgesia
- he is confused by the plasma urate test result – does he have gout even if the urate level was normal?
- he feels frustrated as the foot pain has interrupted his exercise programme; he finds dieting difficult as it is and feels angry with this further set-back to his weight loss programme
- if questioned about the Slighter Lite programme, he tells you it is a very low calorie, low carbohydrate diet; he is getting on well with it, having lost 9 kg in 2 weeks
- he is worried about his raised cholesterol because of his dad's fatal MI 6 months ago.
- he expects the doctor to give him advice about gout, to prescribe analgesia, to advise him on when to repeat his blood tests, and to specify which tests are needed and why

Approach to be taken

A. Data gathering, examination and clinical assessment skills

1. *Define the clinical problem: clarify why the patient has presented today*
   The doctor:
   - makes use of the medical records provided; notices the family history, raised cholesterol, history of gout with a normal serum urate from 2 years ago
   - sees that Mr SF limps in and has a facial expression of pain; he responds to this non-verbal cue immediately, with an appropriate opening sentence such as *"You look as if you have a sore foot"*.
   - asks open questions, such as *"How can I help you today?"* to explore the reasons for Mr SF's presentation today
   - asks closed questions, such as *"On a scale of 1–10, how severe is the pain?"* and *"Where exactly is the pain?"* to clarify details of the foot pain
   - works through a diagnostic sieve to exclude other causes of foot pain (such as trauma or Morton's neuroma) and excludes red flags (septic arthritis or rheumatoid arthritis) by asking *"Are you unwell in yourself? Any temperature symptoms or general body aches?"*
   - elicits how the problem is affecting the patient, his family, or his work: *"Were you able to work with this? How are you managing at home?"*
   - discovers Mr SF's ideas: *"I see from your notes you had gout 2 years ago. Do you think this might be gout?"*
   - discovers Mr SF's concerns: *"What are your concerns about what has happened to you?"*
   - discovers Mr SF's expectations: *"By the end of this consultation, what questions would you like to have had answered?"*
   - discovers Mr SF's health beliefs: *"Am I right in thinking that you doubt the diagnosis of gout because the blood test 2 years ago was normal?"*
   - summarises the problem: *"This sounds like gout, but I would like to examine you. Is that OK?"*

2. *Perform an appropriate physical or mental examination*
   The doctor:
   - performs an appropriate physical examination: number of joints affected, erythema, swelling, tenderness and range of motion; if there is diagnostic doubt, takes the patient's temperature, and explains why the examination is being done
   - performs the examination slickly and with sensitivity
   - explains the examination findings in appropriate language, for example, *"One joint is affected, where the big toe meets the instep; it is red, swollen, warm and painful to touch and move; this is typical of gout"*

B. Clinical management skills

3. *Make an appropriate working diagnosis*
   The doctor:
   - integrates information: recognises conditions associated with gout, such as obesity and hypercholesterolaemia
   - on the basis of probability, makes a clinically sound working diagnosis: understands that serum urate measured during the acute attack may be normal; serum urate should be measured 4–6 weeks after the acute attack has resolved

4. *Explain the problem to the patient using appropriate language*
   The doctor:
   - is patient-centred – uses the patient's ideas and beliefs: *"I can understand why the normal blood test made you doubt the diagnosis of gout, but if the test was done in the middle of the attack, it could be misleading; this looks like gout and we are better off doing the test for gout 6 weeks after this episode settles"*
   - paces the explanation appropriately – *"How do you feel about us sorting the pain out now and doing the blood tests later?"*
   - provides information in adequate chunks and checks understanding at each step – *"Did you know that a diet with lots of meat and alcohol can cause gout?"*; after Mr SF responds, the doctor could then say *"Actually, crash dieting with high protein / low carb. diets can also precipitate gout"*
   - addresses the patient's concerns about his difficulty in losing weight – *"Congratulations on losing 9 kg; this shows motivation and hard work, but do you think this type of eating is sustainable? Could you make smaller changes that you could incorporate into your daily routine?"*
   - addresses the patient's expectations – prescribes an NSAID to be used until 48 hours after the acute attack has resolved – and gives the patient the option: does he want a particular tablet he's used successfully in the past?
   - summarises the problem – *"This looks like gout, which we'll treat using an anti-inflammatory tablet. I'll let you think about whether you want to stop the Slighter Lite diet, but I think it's probably precipitated this attack. We'll confirm if it's gout with a blood test in 6 weeks. It may be useful to repeat your cholesterol and fasting glucose tests at the same time."*
   - actively confirms the patient's understanding of the problem – *"We've discussed quite a lot today. So that I know I've explained properly, could you summarise the plan for me?"*

5. *Provide holistic care and use resources effectively*
   The doctor:
   - makes balanced plans which are either doctor or patient-centred as appropriate – negotiates analgesia, and advises on diet and alcohol intake without hectoring or preaching to the patient

- refers appropriately to the Primary Health Care Team (such as the phlebotomist) and other agencies (such as a dietician) if needed
- practises evidence-based medicine and is informed by national or local guidelines, such as: http://cks.nice.org.uk/gout#!scenario

6. *Prescribe appropriately*
The doctor:

- chooses cost-effective medication, such as diclofenac, indometacin or naproxen, with or without paracetamol and codeine
- discusses medication side effects
- checks the patient's understanding of the medication

7. *Specify the conditions and interval for follow-up*
The doctor:

- safety-nets appropriately: *"If you take the tablets regularly and there is no improvement in the pain within 3 days, could you come back to see me?"*

C. Interpersonal skills: know and treat this patient

8. *Achieve rapport*
The doctor:

- listens attentively, picking up the patient's pain, frustration and uncertainty about the diagnosis, and displays empathy to any adverse psychosocial consequences – *"I can see how you thought this diet would be the solution"*
- uses the patient's ideas about the blood test in his explanations
- addresses the patient's specific concerns about weight management and expectations for acute treatment with appropriate NSAIDs / analgesia

9. *Give the patient the opportunity to be involved in significant management decisions*
The doctor:

- shares thoughts and involves the patient in decisions – *"Any ideas about which painkillers work best for you?"*
- negotiates with the patient – *"I think your low carb. diet may be precipitating this. What do you think? Where can you find more information about the side-effects of this diet?"*
- offers choices or various treatment options – *"I can start with a very potent NSAID and step down, or I could start with a potent one and if it doesn't work, you could combine it with paracetamol. Which option would you prefer?"*
- encourages autonomy and opinions – *"Have a think and decide how you want to manage your weight long term"*

Debrief

Discuss how the doctor could, if needed, improve his performance. In particular, assess whether the doctor:
- established good rapport? If so, which behaviour created rapport? Which statements were particularly useful in achieving rapport?
- presented the patient with appropriate treatment options? Did the doctor risk-assess appropriately prior to prescribing? Did the doctor give appropriate lifestyle advice?
- signposted appropriately? For example, prior to examining, did he ask, *"I'd like to examine you now, is that OK?"*
- summarised appropriately? *"This looks like gout, which we'll treat using an anti-inflammatory tablet. I'll let you think about whether you want to stop the Slighter Lite diet, but I think it's probably precipitated this attack. We'll confirm if it's gout with a blood test in 6 weeks. It may be useful to repeat your cholesterol and fasting glucose tests at the same time."*

If the consultation over-ran:
- was the doctor systematic in his history taking? Did he repeat questions? Did he allow the patient to ramble on uninterrupted?
- were the doctor's explanations simple and non-judgemental?

Revising data gathering

What questions could the doctor ask to discover the patient's ideas, concerns, expectations and health beliefs?
- Ideas: *"What do you think has caused this attack of foot pain?"*
- Concerns: *"Was there anything you were particularly worried about?"*
- Expectations: *"Am I right in thinking you'd like some strong painkillers?"*
- Health beliefs: *"It seems to me that you are slightly confused by the normal blood test result you had two years ago. Shall we discuss how gout is diagnosed in more detail?"*

Relevant literature

http://cks.nice.org.uk/gout#!scenario

tinyurl.com/CS3e-Lc7a (*takes you to* http://arthritis.about.com/od/gout/a/foodstoeat.htm)

Background information

- Gout is associated with serious comorbidity (hypertension (74%), hyperlipidaemia, chronic kidney disease (20%), osteoarthritis, obesity (53%), diabetes (26%), congestive heart failure (11%), and ischaemic heart disease (14%). The increased CV risk is often unrecognised and undertreated.
- The definitive diagnosis of gout requires microscopic identification of monosodium urate crystals but it is more usual to make a clinical diagnosis when the patient has typical features of inflammation, particularly when they affect the first metatarsophalangeal joint. Serum urate values have limited diagnostic value. Serum uric acid concentrations are more important when "treating to target" and are less useful in the diagnosis of gout.
- First-line medical treatment options for acute gout are a non-steroidal anti-inflammatory drug (diclofenac, indometacin, naproxen or etoricoxib 120 mg daily) or low-dose colchicine.
- Long-term management requires full patient education, dealing with any modifiable risk factors (such as overweight or obesity, chronic diuretic intake), and urate-lowering drugs.
- Start allopurinol at a low dose (such as 100 mg daily) and increase gradually with the aim of lowering then maintaining serum urate below 360 µmol/L.

Long case 8 – Achilles tendinosis

Brief to the doctor

Mr GH is a 33 year old man who consults because of an Achilles tendon problem and would like a referral letter to a private physiotherapist.

Patient summary

Name	GH
Date of birth (Age)	33
Social and family history	Married Estate agent Marathon runner
Past medical history	Nil relevant
Current medication	Ibuprofen 400 mg prn

Tasks for the doctor

In this case, the tasks are to:
- clarify and assess the patient's symptoms
- negotiate an appropriate management plan

Brief to the patient – more about the patient

1. Profile:

- GH is a 33 year old estate agent
- married with 2 children aged 7 and 5 years
- he has run the London marathon for charity for the last 5 years and trains 6 days a week
- 4 months ago he started to notice a gradual onset of pain and stiffness in his left mid-calf on waking and this was eased by a hot shower or by walking; this pain has become more severe and it is now interfering with his running

2. He is seeing the doctor today because:

- having researched the subject on the internet and in running magazines, he would like a letter of referral to a private physiotherapist he has located who specialises in sports injuries. He requires the letter in order to recoup the fees on his private health insurance.

3. Additional information:

- If the doctor asks specifically:
  - the onset of symptoms coincided with changing his running route to include hills, as he wanted to increase the workload and decrease the miles covered so that his training was less time-consuming
  - he has had the same running shoes for 7 months – he has always bought anti-pronation running shoes following an assessment in a specialist running footwear shop
- He believes GPs have no expertise in sports medicine and are not sympathetic to the demands of athletes; consequently:
  - he believes this consultation is a waste of time and he is annoyed that he has to see a doctor just to get a referral letter to someone he is paying to see
  - he is not prepared to take any medication or advice from the doctor
  - he is not prepared to be examined
- He is concerned that he will develop a chronic problem that will end his running days completely.

Approach to be taken

A. Data gathering, examination and clinical assessment skills

1. *Define the clinical problem: clarify why the patient has presented today*
   The doctor:
   - reads the patient information provided prior to the consultation
   - asks open questions to explore and clarify Mr GH's symptoms and what he has learned about the condition from his research on the internet and in magazines
   - empathises with his frustration at the restriction of his running schedule
   - asks closed questions to clarify details about possible predisposing factors that might require specific treatment or further referral
   - discovers Mr GH's belief that GPs have no expertise in sports injuries and are not sympathetic to athletes when they are injured
   - uses internal summaries: *"Can I just recap to make sure I have got things right?"*

2. *Performs an appropriate physical or mental examination*
   - In this case, an examination would normally be performed, but the patient refuses to be examined.
   - The need for an examination is explained in appropriate language – *"I would like to examine you in order to ensure that physiotherapy treatment is appropriate before I make a referral."*

B. Clinical management skills

3. *Make an appropriate working diagnosis*
   - The doctor, based on the history, makes a working diagnosis of Achilles tendinopathy.

4. *Explain the problem to the patient using appropriate language*
   The doctor:
   - asks *"What do you know about this problem?"*
   - asks *"Does my explanation make sense? Is there anything else you would like to know?"*
   - explains why private insurers require referral letters

5. *Provide holistic care and use resources effectively*
   - The doctor understands socioeconomic/cultural background: *"It must be very frustrating not being able to run like you used to"*

6. *Prescribe appropriately*
   - The doctor agrees that a physiotherapy referral is appropriate in the first instance and that a physiotherapist with a special interest would be especially beneficial.

7. *Specify the conditions and interval for follow-up*
   - The doctor offers a follow-up appointment if Mr GH does not respond to physiotherapy.

C. Interpersonal skills: know and treat this patient

8. *Achieve rapport*
   The doctor:
   - listens attentively to Mr GH's concerns about his condition
   - explores and clarifies Mr GH's beliefs about GPs' competence in managing sports injuries, but is non-confrontational and non-judgemental
   - understands his request for referral to a specialist physiotherapist
   - shows empathy with Mr GH over his frustration at not being able to train normally and with having to see a doctor for a referral letter

9. *Give the patient the opportunity to be involved in significant management decisions*
   The doctor:
   - actively confirms the patient's understanding of the problem – "*Can I check what you have found out about your problem?*"
   - shares thoughts/involves patient – "*I think you're right to want to see a specialist physio as this problem can be difficult to treat*"

Debrief

Discuss how the doctor could, if needed, improve his performance. In particular, assess how the doctor:

- establishes rapport
- deals with Mr GH's beliefs about GPs' knowledge of sports injuries and sympathy with athletes
- deals with Mr GH's anger at having to consult in order to get a referral letter

Revising data gathering

What questions could the doctor ask to discover the patient's ideas, concerns, expectations and health beliefs?

- Ideas: *"You have done some research for yourself; what have you learned about treatments for your condition?"*
- Concerns: *"Are you worried about the long-term effects of your condition?"*
- Expectations: *"Would you like to ask me about treatments other than physiotherapy?"*
- Health beliefs: *"You don't seem to be very happy about having to see me today, is there a reason for that?"*

Relevant literature

Asplund CA, Best TM. (2013) Achilles tendon disorders. *BMJ*, **346**: f1262. www.bmj.com/content/346/bmj.f1262

Background information

- The Achilles experiences repetitive strain from running, jumping, and sudden acceleration or deceleration, so is susceptible to rupture and degenerative changes.
- Chronic overuse tendon injuries are not caused by inflammation – instead, histology typically shows tissue degeneration and disorganisation.
- Patients with tendinopathy generally describe pain or stiffness in the Achilles 2–6 cm above the calcaneal insertion. Morning stiffness is common, and the pain is usually worse with activity, although it may continue into rest. Less commonly, patients will describe similar symptoms with point tenderness over the insertion of the Achilles on the calcaneus.

Resources for patients

- Kreher JB. Achilles tendinopathy: everything you need to know (and more). What you should know about Achilles tendinopathy to prevent its occurrence and to stop it in its tracks before it stops you. tinyurl.com/CS3e-Lc8a (*takes you to* www.beginnertriathlete.com/...articleid=1694)
- tinyurl.com/CS3e-Lc8b (*takes you to* www.beginnertriathlete.com/...articleid=1313) – video case study on Achilles tendonitis.

Long case 9 – Heel pain

Brief to the doctor

Mr TP is a 28 year old man who presents with a painful left heel. He says that he saw your colleague, Dr Brown, 3 weeks ago and was told he would be referred to physiotherapy. When he phoned the local physiotherapy unit, he was informed that they hadn't received his referral. He still has heel pain.

Patient summary

Name	TP
Date of birth (Age)	28
Social and Family History	Married, with a baby aged 8 weeks
Past medical history	Insurance medical for mortgage 2 years ago – nil of note
Acute medication	Diclofenac 50 mg thrice daily × 60 tablets

Consultation note by Dr Brown (three weeks ago):
'Actuary with gradual onset (4 weeks) L heel pain, worse medially. Started with morning pain and worse after activity. Now unable to finish rugby game over weekend because of 8/10 pain – walked off field. O/E: tender anterior to heel. Impression: typical plantar fasciitis. Plan: diclofenac × 60T and refer to physiotherapy.' (However, there is no referral letter attached to the consultation.)

Tasks for the doctor

In this case, the tasks are to:
- review what has happened since his previous consultation
- decide whether you need to re-examine
- clarify Mr TP's expectations of this consultation and if appropriate, try to meet them

Brief to the patient – more about the patient

1. Profile:

- Mr TP is a 28 year old actuary who works in the city centre
- he commutes to work by train; this is a busy service and occasionally he has to stand for 20 minutes before he can get a seat.
- married with 1 child, aged 8 weeks – she wakes at night and he has to help bottle-feed; he finds the night walking with baby painful
- Mr TP has never been ill before and is worried about his foot; he assumed he would make a quick recovery once he rested the foot for a couple of weeks

2. He is seeing the doctor today because:

- he called the physiotherapy unit to initiate an appointment and found out they hadn't received a referral letter – he wants to know what happened
- his foot still hurts despite rest and ice for 3 weeks – what should he do?
- he was informed by one of his rugby colleagues that an X-ray may be needed to see if he has a heel spur – should he have an X-ray?

3. Additional information:

- if the doctor does not offer him a suitable explanation or apology for what happened to his referral, he becomes increasingly irritated and overtly unhappy
- if the doctor offers him a private referral, he asks if the practice will pay for it as they inadvertently delayed his treatment
- if the doctor offers him a follow-up appointment in the surgery for a steroid injection, he asks for the risks and benefits and chooses not to have this done
- if the doctor gives him advice that will help him while he waits for his NHS physiotherapy appointment, he leaves feeling 'something has been done' and appears slightly appeased

Approach to be taken

A. Data gathering, examination and clinical assessment skills

1. *Define the clinical problem: clarify why the patient has presented today*
   The doctor:
   - reads the patient information provided prior to the consultation and is alerted by the absence of a referral letter
   - asks open questions to explore what Mr TP expects of today's consultation, thereby eliciting a history of the missing physiotherapy referral and on-going left heel pain
   - acknowledges both issues and empathises with his feelings of anxiety and frustration, for example, *"The absence of a referral letter both at the physiotherapy department and here in your notes does not look too promising, does it? I can see how you could be feeling worried about being let down. I don't know what has happened, but I promise you I will look into it and try to resolve this as best I can. Now, I haven't seen you before so I need to ask you some questions so that I can help you."*
   - asks closed questions to clarify details about the current symptoms and treatments tried
   - excludes red flags such as morning stiffness, back and buttock pain, and tenderness in ligament insertions in the extremities (symptoms of Reiter's disease or ankylosing spondylitis – a small minority of these patients present with plantar fasciitis); this set of questions could be signposted by saying, *"To rule out serious illness I need to ask you a few quick questions. Are your joints stiff in the morning; do you have pain in the..."*
   - explores the impact of the symptoms on his work and home life
   - discovers Mr TP's idea that plantar fasciitis should improve within 3 weeks, especially if the foot is rested and NSAIDs taken
   - discovers Mr TP's concern about having to wait even longer for an NHS physiotherapy appointment
   - discovers Mr TP's expectation of practical help in alleviating the pain and aiding recovery

2. *Performs an appropriate physical or mental examination*
   - In this case, because the history and examination findings of the previous consultation are so typical of plantar fasciitis, an examination is not required.
   - However, if examined, the patient is tender in front of the left heel.
   - The foot may have a high arch or may be flat (pes cavus or planus).
   - When walking, the medial arch (observed from behind) drops, creating a flat foot that rolls in.
   - Mr TP does not appear to be overweight.

B. Clinical management skills

3. *Make an appropriate working diagnosis*
   - The doctor, based on the typical history, makes a working diagnosis of plantar fasciitis.

4. *Explain the problem to the patient using appropriate language*
   The doctor:
   - having established that Mr TP knows about plantar fasciitis from his previous consultation, addresses his agenda
   - suggests that his idea that plantar fasciitis resolves quickly may be optimistic: studies show that most cases resolve by 6–12 months, but 5% of patients end up undergoing surgery for plantar fascia release when conservative measures fail: tinyurl.com/CS3e-Lc9a (*takes you to* http://emedicine.medscape.com/article/86143-overview)
   - negotiates a physiotherapy referral; offer to add in a paragraph explaining that the patient had consulted 3 weeks ago and the original referral is missing. Ask Mr TP if he could be available for short notice appointments if other patients cancel and indicate his availability and/or flexibility on the referral document.
   - addresses his expectation of practical advice: discuss footwear, orthotics, silicone heel pads, steroid injections, self massage by rolling the foot on a golf ball, stretching and strengthening exercises: tinyurl.com/CS3e-Lc9b (*takes you to* www.aafp.org/.../p676.html); advise discontinuation of NSAIDs beyond 10 days
   - provides some information on the pros and cons of steroid injection – potential risks include rupture of the plantar fascia and fat pad atrophy
   - provides information on X-rays: plantar fasciitis produces heel spurs; heel spurs do not produce plantar fasciitis, hence, the spur, if present, should not be surgically removed; an X-ray may not add to the management

5. *Provide holistic care and use resources effectively*
   The doctor:
   - practises evidence-based medicine (Thing, J, Maruthappu, M, Rogers, J. (2012) Diagnosis and management of plantar fasciitis in primary care. *British Journal of General Practice*, **62**(601): 443–444)
   - if Mr TP has a good basic understanding of plantar fasciitis, the doctor should build on this knowledge by discussing exercises (foot biomechanics) and self-help treatments

6. *Prescribe appropriately*
   The doctor:
   - checks the patient's understanding of NSAIDs, efficacy and side effects. The doctor suggests appropriate alternative analgesia (paracetamol and/or ibuprofen).

7. *Specify the conditions and interval for follow-up*
   - The doctor offers a follow-up appointment, either to provide a steroid injection or to discuss any issues arising from the physiotherapy.

C. Interpersonal skills: know and treat this patient

8. *Achieve rapport*
   The doctor:
   - listens attentively to Mr TP's opening statements and acknowledges his feelings of fear, anxiety and frustration
   - deals with his anger at the 'lost' referral without placing undue blame on other members of staff
   - displays empathy with regard to the duration of illness and its adverse consequences
   - addresses the patient's specific concerns and expectations and encourages self-help

9. *Give the patient the opportunity to be involved in significant management decisions*
   - The doctor encourages autonomy and opinions – provides him with treatment options, discusses their risks and benefits and facilitates the patient's choice.

Debrief

Discuss how the doctor could, if needed, improve his performance. In particular, assess whether the doctor:
- was able to able to ask the appropriate 'red flag' questions?
- discussed prognosis? If so, was the language used simple and understandable?
- checked the patient's understanding? How did the doctor do this?
- established rapport and defused the patient's anger? If so, how?

If the consultation over-ran, did the doctor:
- re-take a history of the original presentation instead of focusing on what had happened in the interim?
- perform unnecessary examinations or take too long to examine?
- spend too much time placating the 'angry' patient and too little time addressing his need for on-going treatment?

Revising data gathering

What questions could the doctor ask to discover the patient's ideas, concerns, expectations and health beliefs?
- Ideas: *"How long, do you think, it takes for plantar fasciitis to get better?"*
- Concerns: *"The physiotherapy department has not received your referral. What do you suspect has happened?"*
- Expectations: *"You seem to have a good understanding of plantar fasciitis. What specific issues would you like me to address in today's consultation?"*
- Health beliefs: *"You mentioned getting an X-ray to look for heel spurs. Let's discuss this further"*

Relevant literature

Goff, JD, Crawford, R. (2011) Diagnosis and treatment of plantar fasciitis. *American Family Physician*, **84**(6): 676–682.
tinyurl.com/CS3e-Lc9b (*takes you to* www.aafp.org/afp/2011/0915/p676.html)

Background information

Recommended treatments are as follows:
- Biomechanical treatment, including orthotics, footwear modification (such as Rocker-sole shoes), and taping
- Stretching techniques, particularly night splints
- Extracorporeal shock wave therapy, which tends to work only for tendinopathies with calcific change
- Cortisone (or other) injections, such as Botox
- Surgery – surgical division of the plantar fascia.

Long case 10 – Acne

Brief to the doctor

Mr GH is a 24 year old man who consults because he has acne affecting his face and back.

Patient summary

Name	GH
Date of birth (Age)	24
Social and family history	Single Labourer
Past medical history	GP consultations: 14 months ago – *"Acne – face and shoulders. Pustules > comedones. For oxytetracycline 250 mg 2 bd 3/12"* 11 months ago – *"Acne review. No improvement after 3/12 oxytet, add benzoyl peroxide gel. Warned re irritation and bleaching."*
Current medication	None No recorded allergies
Investigations	None

Tasks for the doctor

In this case, the tasks are to:
- review previous medication and try to identify why he has not responded
- identify Mr GH's concerns about his acne and offer support
- prescribe appropriately

Brief to the patient – more about the patient

1. Profile:

- Mr GH is a 24 year old single man
- he works as a labourer on a building site

2. He is seeing the doctor today because:

- he has had acne (spots and blackheads) on his face and back for just over a year and is concerned about the cosmetic appearance
- he saw a GP last year and was given a 3 month course of oxytetracycline without any real benefit; benzoyl peroxide was then added, but again this did not help; he did not bother going back
- he is training to take part in a body building competition – he feels he will not score well in the competition if he is 'spotty'

3. Additional information:

- He was not troubled by acne as a teenager; his voice broke age 11 and he started shaving at 14, by which age he was 6' 1" tall.
- If the doctor asks specifically:
  - he does not come into contact with any chemicals at work
  - for the last 18 months he has been using protein supplements which he buys at the gym
  - most of the other body builders at the gym use steroid tablets and injections
  - he follows a high protein high carbohydrate diet
  - his girlfriend recently split up with him after 4 years together because she was fed up with him always being at the gym and said that he had been become moody and snappy
  - he is not sleeping well; he has no depressive symptoms
- He believes he can train and do well 'naturally'; he refuses to use steroids because he has heard they have long-term effects that are irreversible.
- His trainer has pressured him on several occasions to use steroids. Taking the protein supplements was a compromise that Mr GH complied with to get his trainer 'off his back'.
- He is not aware that some supplements have been reported to contain traces of androgenic-anabolic steroids.
- If the doctor performs an examination:

System	Findings
General	Very well built fit young man No jaundice. No gynaecomastia. Normal body hair
Skin	Comedones and pustules on face, shoulders and back. No scarring or cysts.
Cardiovascular	BP 134/88 (use large cuff)
Abdomen	No enlarged liver No evidence of testicular atrophy

Approach to be taken

A. Data gathering, examination and clinical assessment skills

1. *Define the clinical problem: clarify why the patient has presented today*
   The doctor:
   - reads the patient information provided prior to the consultation
   - asks open questions to explore:
     - whether Mr GH had acne in the past and how it was treated
     - why he is concerned about his acne at this time
     - whether the acne is having any psychosocial effects on him– "*How is this affecting you?*"
     - whether Mr GH has considered that the protein supplements might contain traces of androgenic-anabolic steroids and that this might be the cause of his acne – "*Some sports supplements have been found to contain traces of anabolic steroids and other substances – have you ever wondered about this?*"
   - asks closed questions to:
     - exclude other causes of rashes – "*As a builder, do you come into contact with any irritant chemicals that might cause this?*"
     - be sure that he is not knowingly using androgenic-anabolic steroids or other agents – "*I am sorry, but I have to ask this question because it will affect how we treat your problem. Are you taking any supplements or other substances to enhance your performance or physique?*"
     - assess if he has experienced other possible unwanted effects of androgenic-anabolic steroids – psychological
   - empathises with Mr GH about:
     - the cosmetic effects and having acne occur for the first time at his age rather than in his teens: "*It must be a bit of a shock starting to get acne as an adult rather than as a teenager. How are you coping with that?*"
     - his feelings about androgenic-anabolic steroid use: "*You have heard that anabolic steroids have some serious side-effects, would you like to discuss this?*"

2. *Performs an appropriate physical or mental examination*
   - In this case, a targeted examination is required. A minimally acceptable examination would be, with the patient's shirt removed:
     - examination of the acne to confirm the diagnosis and assess severity
     - a quick visual check to exclude gynaecomastia, loss of body hair, and liver disease stigmata
   - If time permits, a BP check could be done, although this could be deferred to a follow up appointment, given that there are no other signs of anabolic steroid use.
   - The need for an examination should be explained in appropriate language.

B. Clinical management skills

3. *Make an appropriate working diagnosis*
   - The doctor integrates information and makes a working diagnosis of acne probably secondary to androgenic-anabolic steroid use.
   - This is a clinically sound hypothesis with an appropriate use of probability.

4. *Explain the problem to the patient using appropriate language*
   The doctor:
   - having established Mr GH's feelings about drugs, sensitively explains that some protein supplements have been reported to contain androgenic-anabolic steroids – *"If I were to say to you that some supplements have been reported to contain anabolic steroids, how would you feel?"*
   - explains that acne is a reported unwanted effect of androgenic-anabolic steroids
   - provides information on androgenic-anabolic steroids to include unwanted effects
   - advises Mr GH that the unwanted effects are largely reversible if androgenic-anabolic steroid use is stopped
   - uses chunking and checking of information to evaluate Gary's understanding: *"I have given you a lot of unexpected information, before I examine you, can I just check that I have explained things clearly?"*

5. *Provide holistic care and use resources effectively*
   The doctor:
   - builds on Mr GH's health beliefs to identify management options – *"You've told me that you are against drugs, would you be happy to stop using the supplements and see if the problem goes away?"*
   - understands socioeconomic/cultural background – *"Are you concerned that stopping the supplements might affect your chances in the competition?"*
   - discusses with Mr GH whether to perform blood tests to look for biochemical effects of androgenic-anabolic steroids – *"It is possible that you may have been taking a supplement that contains steroids and that this is the cause of your acne. We have talked about some of the side effects of these. Would you like to have a blood test to check whether there are any signs of other side effects?"*

6. *Prescribe appropriately*
   - The doctor agrees an appropriate management plan with the patient to include:
     - that Mr GH should stop taking the protein supplements and be reviewed in a month to see if his acne had improved
     - having blood tests – FBC, U&Es, LFTs, fasting glucose and fasting lipids

7. *Specify the conditions and interval for follow-up*
   - The doctor arranged a follow-up appointment to monitor progress of the acne and review the blood test results.

C. Interpersonal skills: know and treat this patient

8. *Achieve rapport*
   The doctor:
   - listens attentively
   - follows up verbal and non-verbal cues – *"You mentioned body-building, I know that some body builders use special supplements to improve their performance..."*
   - sensitively explores and clarifies Mr GH's supplement use and his feelings about androgenic-anabolic steroids
   - places the problem in a psychosocial context – how it affects patient/relationships: *"You mentioned that your girlfriend said you were moody and snappy, was this just with her?"*
   - is non-judgemental about Mr GH's use of protein supplements
   - empathises with Mr GH about getting acne in adult life

9. *Give the patient the opportunity to be involved in significant management decisions*
   The doctor:
   - actively confirms patient's understanding of the problem – *"Is there anything else you would like to ask?"*
   - shares thoughts with the patient that the protein supplements may be causing the acne
   - encourages autonomy by building on Mr GH's ideas and concerns about taking anabolic steroids to agree a management plan

Debrief

Discuss how the doctor could, if needed, improve his performance. In particular, assess how the doctor:

- established rapport and identified Mr GH's beliefs about androgenic-anabolic steroid use
- raised the possibility of the supplements containing androgenic-anabolic steroids and that this might be the cause of his acne

Revising data gathering

What questions could the doctor ask to discover the patient's ideas, concerns, expectations and health beliefs?

- Ideas: "*I understand that you are surprised that you have started getting acne at your age, do you have any ideas why this has happened now?*"
- Concerns: "*Are you concerned that you might have other side effects of anabolic steroids?*"
- Expectations: "*Would you like to have some blood tests to see if there are any signs of other steroid side effects?*"
- Health beliefs: "*You said that you are worried about the long-term effects of androgenic-anabolic steroids, would you like to discuss this?*"

Relevant literature

Bahrke MS, Yesalis CE. (2002) *Performance-Enhancing Substances in Sport and Exercise.* Human Kinetics, Champaign Illinois.

World Anti-Doping Agency (WADA) website: www.wada-ama.org
WADA Athlete guide is available at this website in twelve languages:
tinyurl.com/CS3-Lc10a (*takes you to* www.wada-ama.org/.../athlete-reference-guide-to-2015-code-online-version)

Background information

- Consider an oral antibiotic combined with either a topical retinoid or benzoyl peroxide if there is acne on the back or shoulders that is particularly extensive or difficult to reach, or if there is a significant risk of scarring or substantial pigment change.
  - Oral tetracycline, oxytetracycline, doxycycline, or lymecycline are first-line options. Erythromycin is an alternative if tetracyclines are poorly tolerated or contraindicated (such as in pregnancy). Minocycline is not recommended.
  - Do not prescribe an oral antibiotic alone.
  - Do not combine a topical and an oral antibiotic.
  - Oral antibiotics should be limited to the shortest possible period, and discontinued when further improvement of acne is unlikely.
- Arrange follow-up after about 6–8 weeks to review the effectiveness and tolerability of treatment, and the person's compliance with the treatment.
- If there has been some response, continue treatment for up to 6 months.

Investigation	Potential abnormality in steroid use
Associated with anabolic steroid use	
Testosterone: epitestosterone ratio*	Elevated (>4:1)
Gonadotropins LH and FSH	Suppressed
IGF-1†	Elevated
Indicators of anabolic steroid complications	
Prolactin	Elevated
Full blood count	Platelet aggregation and erythropoiesis
Serum glucose	Elevated
Urea and electrolytes	Elevated Na+, depressed K+
Lipid profile	Elevated LDL, low HDL
Liver function tests‡	Cholestatic picture, elevated alanine transaminase‡
Creatine kinase‡	Elevated in muscle damage, consider rhabdomyolysis
γ-glutamyltransferase‡	Elevated in liver damage
Hepatitis and HIV infection	Positive if needle sharing
ECG and echocardiogram if suspect long term use or cardiac symptoms	Cardiomegaly or ischaemic heart disease

LH = luteinising hormone. FSH = follicle stimulating hormone. IGF-1 = Insulin-like growth factor 1. LDL = low density lipoprotein. HDL = high density lipoprotein. ECG = electrocardiogram.
*May not be routinely available.
†Marker of growth hormone secretion.
‡Elevated alanine transaminase and creatine kinase may be due to heavy weight training; γ-glutamyltransferase is a more sensitive marker of hepatic function.

Reproduced from *BMJ*; Brooks, J.H.M., Ahmad, I. and Easton, G., Investigations to consider in suspected or confirmed use of anabolic steroids; 355:i5023, 2016, with permission from BMJ Publishing Group Ltd.

Long case 11 – Post-partum problems

Brief to the doctor

Mrs PH is a 32 year old woman who is added to the end of your clinic as a telephone consultation. You call her back on the number supplied. Mrs PH saw the practice nurse 4 days ago for blood tests.

Patient summary

Name	PH
Date of birth (Age)	34
Social and Family History	Married with two children Her son was born 10 days ago
Past medical history	Heartburn during pregnancy
Current medication	Gaviscon as required

Consultation note by practice nurse (four days ago):
'Discharged from labour ward but advised to have FBC taken as loss of 850 ml blood. Is feeling light-headed but not SOB. Blood taken from L cubital fossa using aseptic technique. Patient advised to call surgery for results in 3–5 days.'

Blood tests	Tests were done four days ago
Hb	10.5 g/dl (12–15)
MCV	97 (83–105)
White cell count	6.67 (4–11)
Differential count	no abnormalities
Platelet count	285 (150–400)

Tasks for the doctor

In this case, the tasks are to:
- clarify, with attention to auditory cues, Mrs PH's reason(s) for calling
- take a detailed history
- actively confirm that the patient understands the treatment plan

Brief to the patient – more about the patient

1. Profile:

- Mrs PH is a 34 year old woman who is currently on maternity leave; her baby boy was born 10 days ago
- she is married and has an older daughter, aged 6
- Mrs PH wants the results of her blood tests; she was also advised by the health visitor to tell you about the 'clot' she has passed

2. She is calling the doctor today because:

- she would like to know the results of her recent blood tests and whether treatment is needed
- the health visitor advised her to tell the GP about the clot she passed: two days ago, she passed one small clot vaginally – it was the size of a 50 pence coin; the clot did not seem to contain any tissue and there have not been other clots or smelly discharge or abdominal pain
- when asked about the birth, she tells you that her waters broke at 2 pm, her labour progressed quickly, her baby was born by NVD at 10 pm, but she was then taken to theatre for a manual removal of placenta, hence the 850 ml loss of blood; she cannot remember if the she was given antibiotics intravenously at the time of the procedure and she was not given antibiotic tablets after the manual removal
- she feels well in herself and has not had fever or rigors
- her main concern is that treatments may interfere with her breastfeeding; she has had a few problems with breastfeeding, which is why she is seeing the health visitor for advice – she wants to breastfeed and would prefer to avoid formula milk if at all possible; she is wary of antibiotics, particularly if antibiotics pass into breast milk and give the baby diarrhoea, resulting in further weight loss
- she expects advice: what should she do about her blood results and her bleeding?

3. Additional information:

- if the doctor discusses an iron-rich diet, she says that she eats meat, bran, baked beans, etc. and has no problem avoiding tea and coffee with meals
- if the doctor suggests iron tablets, she says she has not had problems with iron tablets in the past – she expects the doctor to make arrangements for the prescription
- if you suggest a wait and see policy, she expects to be told when to seek your advice again
- if you suggest that she comes in to see a GP, she wants to know if she needs to attend today as arranging childcare for her 6 year old may be difficult

Approach to be taken

A. Data gathering, examination and clinical assessment skills

1. *Define the clinical problem: clarify why the patient has telephoned today*
   The doctor:
   - reads the patient information provided prior to the consultation and notes that Mrs HP lost 850 ml of blood during birth and now has an Hb of 10.6 g/dl
   - telephones Mrs HP on the number provided; he introduces himself and establishes the identity of the patient – if someone else answers, he asks to speak to the patient because a first-hand history is usually more reliable
   - clarifies the nature of the problem and understands exactly what the patient is requesting today; one approach is *"I see from your notes you recently gave birth. Congratulations! I also see that you had some blood tests done a few days ago. What can I do for you today?"*
   - asks open questions to explore the two issues raised by the patient, such as *"How are you feeling now?"* or *"Tell me more about the clots"*
   - asks closed questions to clarify details about the post-partum bleeding: fever, rigors, feeling unwell, racing pulse, risk factors for endometritis, such as a manual removal of placenta; by asking about current infection, the doctor systematically excludes red flags signalling the need for review or referral
   - empathises with her difficulties in breastfeeding and elicits her concerns regarding treatments that may interfere with breastfeeding
   - elicits her expectations for advice regarding her two issues, namely anaemia and post-partum bleeding

2. *Performs an appropriate physical or mental examination*
   - In this case, an examination is not required. The difficulty with telephone triage is the ability to make management decisions in the absence of visual cues.

B. Clinical management skills

3. *Make an appropriate working diagnosis*
   - The doctor, based on the history, makes a working diagnosis of (1) anaemia due to blood loss at delivery, and (2) the possibility of secondary post-partum haemorrhage (PPH) due to endometrial infection.

4. *Explain the problem to the patient using appropriate language*
   The doctor:
   - addresses Mrs PH's agenda: what does Mrs PH know about dietary treatments for anaemia / iron tablets / fluids that reduce iron absorption? The doctor may explain why he is concerned about the PV bleeding – that it could be a warning sign of 'hidden infection in the womb'

- gives the information about PPH in digestable chunks: a severe case of PPH would have more bleeding or purulent lochia, the patient would feel unwell (like flu), have a racing pulse, feel flushed and feverish, with sweating that wets the clothes; the patient's understanding is checked at each step
- addresses Mrs PH's concerns: an iron-rich diet, with or without iron tablets, is unlikely to interfere with breastfeeding; further assessment of the vaginal bleed may be needed in the form of a pelvic examination – she may not want her 6 year old daughter present during this examination (or the curtains could be drawn around the bed for privacy) – the assessment could take place within the next few days, at her convenience; however, if symptoms of severe infection develop, she needs to see a doctor urgently
- 'prescribes' an iron-rich diet and negotiates prescription of iron tablets according to Mrs PH's preferences

5. *Provide holistic care and use resources effectively*
The doctor:
- manages both problems (anaemia and PV bleeding) in accordance with national or local guidelines
- checks that there is agreement and understanding with what is proposed
- does not waste time addressing the breastfeeding issue if Mrs CC is happy with the advice she has received from the health visitor – the time is better spent addressing her concerns about anaemia and PV bleeding

6. *Prescribe appropriately*
The doctor:
- is aware of national and local guidelines – tinyurl.com/CS3e-Lc11a (*takes you to* www.nice.org.uk/guidance/CG37/...)
- if prescribing, discusses how iron tablets are taken and the commonly experienced side effects

7. *Specify the conditions and interval for follow-up*
The doctor:
- arranges the follow-up appointment for the pelvic examination
- outlines the red flag symptoms; if these symptoms develop, Mrs PH should seek urgent care (i.e safety-nets)
- summarises, for example, with *"Just to recap, we've agreed that you will eat more red meat and cornflakes and avoid tea and coffee with meals. Your husband will collect the prescription for iron tablets and you will take one tablet daily with orange juice. You will keep an eye on your vaginal bleeding. If it is settling you will see me for an examination at your convenience in the next few days. If you develop a temperature, more bleeding, or start to feel unwell, you will ring back and I will see you as an emergency appointment. Are you happy with these arrangements?"*

C. Interpersonal skills: know and treat this patient

8. *Achieve rapport*

   The doctor:
   - listens attentively to Mrs PH's request for advice, does not interrupt unnecessarily, and maintains the flow of conversation
   - questions in a systematic manner, taking care to deal with one issue at a time
   - is sensitive in his queries and ensures that the conversation does not sound like an interrogation
   - understands the patient's request for advice and refrains from making comments such as *"I don't know why the health visitor didn't sort this out herself!"*
   - displays empathy to her predicament – *"I can understand why you'd prefer to avoid any tablets that interfere with the breastfeeding routine you've worked so hard to establish. Let me reassure you that iron tablets will not affect the feeding."*
   - is alert to the possibility of PPH in someone who has had a manual removal of the placenta; however, he does not alarm the patient unduly

9. *Give the patient the opportunity to be involved in significant management decisions*
   - The doctor encourages autonomy and opinions – provides the patient with information on diet and iron tablets and allows her to choose her own treatment; provides sufficient information on why a pelvic examination may be needed and Mrs PH is able to make an appointment that fits in with her childcare

Debrief

Discuss how the doctor could, if needed, improve his performance. In particular, assess whether the doctor:

- established rapport on the telephone? If so, how?
- established the patient's reasons for calling? If so, how?
- dealt with Mrs PH's specific concerns in a systematic manner? If so, how?
- discussed the red flags for PPH in a non-alarmist manner?
- summarised and checked understanding?

If the consultation over-ran, did the doctor:

- interrupt unnecessarily?
- get side-tracked by other issues, such as breastfeeding, that Mrs PH was happy to leave to the health visitor?
- repeat some explanations and reassurances?

Revising data gathering

What questions could the doctor ask to discover the patient's ideas, concerns, expectations and health beliefs?

- Ideas: *"Do you have any ideas on how anaemia (low blood counts) is treated?"*
- Concerns: *"Regarding the clot, did you have any worries about what might be happening?"*
- Expectations: *"It seems to me that you want a treatment that does not interfere with your breastfeeding. Do I understand you correctly?"*
- Health beliefs: *"You sound as if you suspect that something is not quite right if you pass a clot a week after delivering. Let's talk about this for a moment."*

Relevant literature

tinyurl.com/CS3e-Lc11b (*takes you to* www.weightlossresources.co.uk/.../iron_rich_food.htm)

tinyurl.com/CS3e-Lc11c (*takes you to* www.bsg.org.uk/.../bsg_ida_2011.pdf)

Background information

The commonest causes of PPH (blood loss >500 ml) are uterine atony, retained placenta or lacerations / trauma of the birth canal.

Risk factors for PPH:
- History of previous PPH
- Family history of PPH (women with a sister who had a PPH may have an increased risk of PPH themselves)
- Advanced maternal age
- Fibroids
- Hypertensive disorders
- Obesity
- Chorioamnionitis
- Placenta praevia
- Prolonged or augmented labour
- Macrosomia.

Offer pregnant women with haemoglobin <110 g/L iron supplementation - it reduces the risk of anaemia and low birth weight.

Long case 12 – Relative with bowel cancer

Brief to the doctor

Mr KL is a 20 year old man who presents in a routine surgery. He has registered as a temporary resident as he is in his first year at university. He has come home because his father has recently had surgery for bowel cancer at the age of 44 years. He has asked to talk about genetic screening for bowel cancer with a doctor. Mr KL saw one of your partners last year, just before he left to go to university, when he had noticed some blood on the toilet paper for a few days, but he was told not to worry.

Patient summary

Name	KL
Date of birth (Age)	20
Social and family history	Student Father diagnosed with cancer of the bowel 2 months ago
Past medical history	GP consultation: 1 year ago – "*c/o fresh blood on toilet paper when he wipes – 4 days, none in pan. Stool normal but has been straining a bit. Well in self. No pain. Prob pile. Reassured, told to return if continues.*"
Current medication	None
Investigations	None

Tasks for the doctor

In this case, the tasks are to:
- confirm details of his father's diagnosis and any advice given for relatives by the hospital consultant, while respecting KL's father's right to confidentiality; as a result discuss whether Mr KL should be referred for genetic advice and screening
- explore Mr KL's concerns about his rectal bleeding last year
- discuss symptoms and factors linked with bowel cancer, including genetics; discuss any lifestyle changes Mr KL may like to make

Brief to the patient – more about the patient

1. Profile:

- Mr KL is a 20 year old Sports Science student
- he lives in a hall of residence but tends not to eat there as he often goes to the gym in the evenings and so has takeaways or Pot Noodles in the evenings
- he saw one of the GPs in this practice a year ago because he had had some rectal bleeding and was told he probably had a pile and need not worry. He has had a couple of episodes of fresh blood on the paper since then. His health is excellent – he feels well and has not lost weight.
- his father had rectal bleeding 6 months ago and saw the same partner KL saw last year and the father was also told he probably had piles and not to worry – he then saw another partner and was referred to the hospital 2 months ago. Mr KL's father has told him that he had a 'Stage 2' tumour. His father has had a right hemicolectomy and is going to have chemotherapy.
- Mr KL is angry that his father was not referred earlier by your partner and concerned that he had the same symptoms and was also 'fobbed off' without an examination
- Mr KL believes that lifestyle has a major effect on health and is very open to health promotion advice – he feels guilty that he has neglected his own diet
- he has not looked up bowel cancer on the internet yet as he has not had time, but intends to do so

2. He is seeing the doctor today because:

- he wants information on the genetics of bowel cancer and advice on whether he should have screening; he would like to discuss what screening tests are possible and their accuracy
- he would like to be reassured about his own rectal bleeding and would like to be told exactly what the cause is – he feels he should be examined and referred to a specialist
- he wants advice on what preventive measures he can take

3. Additional information:

- If the doctor examines him:

System	Findings
General	Well. No evidence of weight loss No pallor
Abdomen	Soft. No tenderness No masses or organomegaly
Rectal examination	Perianal skin – NAD. No external piles/skin tags Empty rectum. No masses felt. No blood on glove

Approach to be taken

A. Data gathering, examination and clinical assessment skills

1. Define the clinical problem: clarify why the patient has presented today
The doctor:
- reads the patient information provided prior to the consultation
- asks open questions to clarify details of:
  - Mr KL's father's condition – *"I haven't got your father's records, tell me about him."*
  - Mr KL's concerns for himself – *"You seem concerned that you have the same symptoms as your father?"*
  - Mr KL's request for information on genetic screening – *"What do you know about screening for bowel cancer?"*
  - Mr KL's knowledge about causes of the condition
- asks closed questions to clarify:
  - details of Mr KL's own symptoms to exclude red flag symptoms signalling the need for review or referral
  - what advice, if any, the hospital has given about screening the rest of the family
- uses internal summaries – *"Can I just check I've got things right…"*

2. Performs an appropriate physical or mental examination
- In this case, an examination is required to address the patient's concerns.
- The examination should be explained in appropriate language – *"I need to examine your abdomen and then do an internal examination with a finger."*
- A targeted examination should be performed – abdomen and RE.

B. Clinical management skills

3. Make an appropriate working diagnosis
- The doctor, based on the history and examination, makes a working diagnosis of haemorrhoidal bleeding.
- This is a clinically sound hypothesis and makes an appropriate use of probability.

4. Explain the problem to the patient using appropriate language
The doctor:
- explains the likely cause of Mr KL's symptoms
- addresses Mr KL's agenda:
  - that he should be referred to ensure he does not have cancer
  - discusses factors associated with bowel cancer pertinent to him including diet and genetics: *"What do you know about causes of bowel cancer?"*
  - discusses screening for bowel cancer: *"Do you know much about screening for bowel cancer?"*

- addresses Mr KL's concerns about the management of his father in a non-judgemental way and respecting his father's confidentiality

5. *Provide holistic care and use resources effectively*
   The doctor:
   - practises evidence-based medicine using national guidelines – NICE (2015) *Suspected cancer: recognition and referral.* NG12 – tinyurl.com/CS3e-Lc12a (*takes you to* www.nice.org.uk/guidance/ng12/...)
   - uses Mr KL's health beliefs to reinforce advice about preventive measures he could take – "*You seem to be keen on preventing cancers, would you like to discuss things you might be able to do to decrease your risks?*"
   - respects his father's right to confidentiality – "*I am afraid I can't discuss details of your father's case without his permission. Can I suggest you discuss your concerns with your family to see if they share your feelings?*"
   - advises Mr KL about the complaints procedure – "*Would you like me to give you details of how to make a complaint, if you and your family decide to do so?*"

6. *Prescribe appropriately*
   The doctor:
   - chooses to advise Mr KL about diet rather than provide local treatments (haemorrhoid creams) for the management of his symptoms
   - writes to Mr KL's father's consultant to ask if Mr KL should also be referred for screening as his father had developed bowel cancer before the age of 45, with a copy to Mr KL's GP at university for information

7. *Specify the conditions and interval for follow-up*
   The doctor:
   - offers a follow-up appointment to discuss any issues arising from Mr KL's own symptoms, lifestyle change and his father's condition
   - checks understanding: "*Just to check that I have explained things clearly, can you tell me what we have agreed to do today?*"

C. Interpersonal skills: know and treat this patient

8. *Achieve rapport*
   The doctor:
   - listens attentively to Mr KL's concerns about:
     - his father's condition and perceived delayed referral
     - his own symptoms and his risk of developing bowel cancer in the future
   - explores and clarifies Mr KL's health beliefs and concerns – that lifestyle contributes to maintaining health
   - understands his request for information on screening and genetic counselling
   - is non-judgemental about the patient's ideas on his father's management, but expresses sympathy with Mr KL's feelings and upset

9. *Give the patient the opportunity to be involved in significant management decisions*
   The doctor:
   - actively confirms the patient's understanding of the problem: "*Does my explanation of the likely cause of your symptoms sound reasonable to you?*"
   - balances plans – doctor/patient centred as appropriate – "*I don't think I need to refer you about your bleeding at the moment, but agree it would be sensible to check with the hospital whether your father had one of the sorts of cancer that might have a genetic component, in which case you will need to be referred*"

Debrief

Discuss how the doctor could, if needed, improve his performance. In particular, assess how the doctor:

- obtained information about Mr KL's father's cancer to enable him to answer Mr KL's questions. Did he get all the necessary information from Mr KL or could he have consulted the father's medical records? What are the issues relating to discussing his father's records with Mr KL?
- dealt with Mr KL's rectal bleeding symptoms. Was an examination appropriate or necessary? Should a chaperone be offered?
- dealt with Mr KL's anger over his partner's advice to both Mr KL and his father
- gained Mr KL's trust

Revising data gathering

What questions could the doctor ask to discover the patient's ideas, concerns, expectations and health beliefs?

- Ideas: *"You seem to be angry about the advice the other doctor gave you and your father; would you like to discuss that?"*
- Concerns: *"Are you worried that you might develop bowel cancer at some time in the future?"*
- Expectations: *"You said you were unhappy that my partner didn't examine you last year; would you prefer to be examined today?"* and *"I understand your anxiety about your own symptoms and why you would like an exact diagnosis, how were you hoping I would help with those today?"*
- Health beliefs: *"Being fit and healthy is important to you; would you like to discuss things you can do that might decrease your chances of developing bowel cancer?"*

Once the doctor has gathered sufficient information, how could he summarise the problem for the patient?

- *"We have discussed a lot of things today, can I just summarise them to make sure I have covered all the things you wanted and that we have agreed on what to do about them all?"*
- *"Are you happy with what we have covered or do you have any questions or concerns?"*

Relevant literature

Hamilton W (2015) Suspected cancer (part 2 – adults): reference tables from updated NICE guidance. *BMJ*, **350**: h3044.

Jones R, Latinovic R, Charlton J, Gulliford MC. (2007) Alarm symptoms in early diagnosis of cancer in primary care: cohort study using General Practice Research Database. *BMJ*, **334**: 1040–1044.

Department of Health (2000) *Referral guidelines for suspected cancer.*

NICE (2005) *Referral guidelines for suspected cancer*, CG27: www.nice.org.uk/Guidance/CG27

Background information

If the patient has just a single first-degree relative with a history of bowel cancer that he/she developed over the age of 50, then there is no need for bowel cancer screening for relatives. Reassure the patient that the risk of bowel cancer is low (smaller than 1 in 12 and therefore not significantly increased over that of the general population), encourage participation in the National Bowel Cancer Screening Programme when eligible, and advise on red flag symptoms for bowel cancer that should trigger the patient to seek further advice, such as change in bowel habit, rectal bleeding, abdominal pain or mass, unexplained weight loss, or unexplained tiredness, dizziness or breathlessness.

Patients with stronger family history or with a family history of colorectal cancer in a first-degree relative under the age of 50 may warrant referral for colonoscopic screening.

It is important to suspect a genetic syndrome associated with increased risk of colorectal cancer and refer for specialist follow-up and genetic counselling if:
- There is a family history consistent with an autosomal-dominant cancer syndrome, especially if there is more than one close relative affected at a young age (i.e. under the age of 50 years)
- There are other clinical features consistent with a genetic polyposis syndrome either in the patient or a close relative of the patient
- A colorectal cancer susceptibility gene is identified in the patient or any first-degree relative.

Long case 13 – Food poisoning

Brief to the doctor

Mr EJ is a 32 year old man who consulted your colleague, Dr Brown 5 days ago. The microbiology laboratory telephoned the practice nurse this morning to relay the results of Mr EJ's stool sample: campylobacter was isolated. The nurse added Mr EJ to your appointment list for you to telephone him with the results.

Patient summary

Name	EJ
Date of birth (Age)	32
Social and Family History	Unmarried; works as an airline steward
Past medical history	Low back pain 6 months ago Poor sleep pattern 2 years ago
Medication	None

Dr Brown's consultation (5 days ago)
'Diarrhoea symptoms: frequent, loose motions. Fresh blood from piles and no mucus. Passing watery stool every 1–2 hours. Crampy, abdominal pain – using NSAIDs and paracetamol. Recent travel to Jordan and Germany; stayed in hotels. Ate egg sandwich at Frankfurt airport. Had salmonella age 17. O/E: hydrated, slightly dry lips. Generalised abdominal tenderness. No guarding. T 37.3°C. Plan: get stool samples × 2. Use Imodium only if diarrhoea is interrupting sleep. Not due back at work for a few days.'

Tasks for the doctor

In this case, the tasks are to:
- contact Mr EJ with his results
- review his symptoms
- provide appropriate occupational advice

Brief to the patient – more about the patient

1. Profile:

- Mr EJ is a 32 year old man who works as a steward for a budget airline
- he is unmarried and lives alone; he has had several relationships with partners of the same sex. His last HIV test at the GUM clinic 3 months ago, after the break-up of his most recent relationship, was negative. He has used condoms since.
- Mr EJ feels ill and is worried about the abdominal cramp he is experiencing with this bout of food poisoning.

2. When the surgery contacts him, he updates them on his illness:

- the diarrhoea has improved but he does not feel completely well
- he passes two to three loose, not watery, stools daily and is now able to sleep through the night; he did not use any tablets to reduce stool frequency – he drank fluids to rehydrate and now tolerates bland food. He does not have nausea or vomiting.
- he still experiences generalised stomach cramp, unrelated to meals, but the cramp is not as severe (3/10) nor does it last as long (10 minutes) compared to 5 days ago
- he has been recuperating at home. However, he is due to fly to Spain on the early flight tomorrow and thinks he feels well enough to undertake the short-haul. He works several flights for the next 3 days after which he meets with friends in Spain where a party is planned.
- he is shocked to hear about the positive campylobacter result; he expected the cultures to be negative, and he wants to know if further treatment is needed
- he expects to return to work tomorrow – is this OK? As a steward, one of his duties is to sell packaged food and beverages on flights.
- does he need to inform work about his results?
- with regard to the party, is he OK to drink alcohol?
- Mr EJ is a chatty man and one of the difficulties in this case is to remain focused on the relevant medical issues

3. Additional information:

- if the doctor does not prescribe antibiotics, he wants to know if there could be complications later on?
- should he give a stool sample at a later date to check for eradication?
- if the doctor prescribes antibiotics, he wants to know if he can return to work within 24 hours – presumably he won't be infectious then?
- this is his 2nd bowel infection – is there something predisposing him to bowel infections? Is there anything he can do to prevent getting infections?

Approach to be taken

A. Data gathering, examination and clinical assessment skills

1. *Define the clinical problem: inform the patient of the results and clarify the issues a positive result has for him*
   The doctor:
   - reads the patient notes provided prior to the telephone consultation and thinks about what information he needs to obtain from Mr EJ
   - telephones Mr EJ on the number provided and introduces himself; he establishes the identity of the caller / patient and speaks to the patient directly
   - signposts or structures the consultations, for example, says *"Mr EJ, I have the results of your stool sample. Before we discuss these, I'd like to ask you some questions."*
   - asks open questions to explore how Mr EJ is feeling at the moment and, if there has been an improvement, what has improved and what helped him to feel better
   - asks closed questions to clarify details about fever, pain, diarrhoea (frequency, consistency, presence of blood or mucus) since he was last seen
   - asks about red flag symptoms, namely feeling very unwell, having a high temperature (sepsis or systemic illness), passing more than eight stools per day, being ill for longer than 1 week, being immunocompromised, change in bowel habit, rectal bleeding, weight loss or dehydration
   - empathises with the pain and disruption the diarrhoea has caused to Mr EJ's usual routine; clarifies the impact the illness has had on his family and work. The doctor is alert to the fact that Mr EJ is a food handler.
   - discovers Mr EJ's idea that his illness is a mild, self-limiting case of food poisoning, his expectation of returning to work as an airline steward tomorrow, and his concern about whether work should be informed about a positive campylobacter result

2. *Performs an appropriate physical or mental examination*
   - In this case, an examination is not required.

B. Clinical management skills

3. *Make an appropriate working diagnosis*
   - The doctor, based on the history, makes a working diagnosis of improving campylobacter diarrhoea. In the absence of red flag symptoms, antibiotics are not indicated. However, this needs to be balanced against his status as a food handler who, if not given antibiotics, may continue to shed organisms in the stool for up to 4 weeks. Infection usually occurs via infected food or

water; person-to-person transmission via the faeco-oral route is rare. In addition, Mr EJ handles packaged food so the risk of transmission is further reduced.

4. *Explain the problem to the patient using appropriate language*
   The doctor:
   - having established that Mr EJ is improving, informs him of his microbiology results
   - provides him with information about the natural history of campylobacter gastroenteritis and possible treatments: rehydration (200 ml after each loose stool), antibiotics in severe cases (erythromycin or ciprofloxacin), avoid antimotility drugs, and probiotics may help to reduce the duration of diarrhoea by 1 day
   - provides some occupational advice: all workers, including food handlers, are advised to return to work 48 hours after the last episode of diarrhoea
   - addresses Mr EJ's specific questions about possible complications (15% develop irritable bowel syndrome post-infection)

5. *Provide holistic care and use resources effectively*
   The doctor:
   - practises evidence-based medicine that is informed by national or local guidelines
   - informs Mr EJ about camplylobacter being a notifiable disease (search for "notifiable diseases" on www.hpa.org.uk)
   - if Mr EJ does not raise the issue of a 'sick note', the doctor (time permitting) may wish to inform him that 'fit notes' are issued for sickness absences lasting more than 6 days
   - some companies offer flexible working patterns and if the patient is unable to attend work (e.g. with diarrhoea), then some work, especially if computer or internet based, can be done from home; patients are encouraged to liaise directly with their occupational health or human resources departments

6. *Prescribe appropriately*
   - The doctor is aware of national and local guidelines when making a decision on prescribing: tinyurl.com/CS3e-Lc13a (*takes you to* https://cks. nice.org.uk/diarrhoea-adults-assessment...)

7. *Specify the conditions and interval for follow-up*
   The doctor:
   - discusses the 'red flag' symptoms and advises the patient to consult if these develop
   - if sick certification advice is provided, the advice is in line with national guidance

C. Interpersonal skills: know and treat this patient

8. *Achieve rapport*
   The doctor:
   - listens attentively to Mr EJ's account of his current symptoms and displays empathy to its adverse impact on his life
   - understands his request for information on the natural history and possible treatments of campylobacter as the patient knows very little about this infection
   - uses his ideas about self-limiting illness in explanations
   - addresses his specific concerns about what to tell work and his expectations of when to resume air stewarding duties

9. *Give the patient the opportunity to be involved in significant management decisions*
   The doctor:
   - discusses the pros and cons of antibiotic and probiotic treatments and negotiates with the patient
   - encourages patient autonomy by providing him with enough information so that he feels able to discuss work issues with his company

Debrief

Discuss how the doctor could, if needed, improve his performance. In particular, assess whether the doctor:

- asked questions in a systematic and structured manner? If so, how?
- asked about red flag symptoms? If so, how long did this take? Was this sign-posted? (for example, did the doctor preface his questions with *"I need to ask some questions to rule out serious illness – do you have any of the following?"*)
- discussed the evidence base for appropriate treatments?
- provided appropriate occupational medicine advice?

If the consultation over-ran, did the doctor:

- take too long to ask the red flag questions?
- spend too much time on small-talk?
- attempt to reduce consulting time by offering the patient a face-to-face appointment instead? This option may not be the most efficient use of resources.

Revising data gathering

What questions could the doctor ask to discover the patient's ideas, concerns, expectations and health beliefs?

- Ideas: *"What, in your experience, has been the best way of dealing with food poisoning? What's worked, and not worked, for you in the past?"*
- Concerns: *"Is there anything in particular that concerns you about this positive campylobacter result?"*
- Expectations: *"It seems to me that we have discussed your symptoms and treatment. However, I suspect you may have some questions about work. Are there any questions in particular you'd like me to answer?"*
- Health beliefs: *"You suspect that because this is your second episode of gut infection, you may be predisposed to gut infections. Let's talk about this for a moment."*

Relevant literature

tinyurl.com/CS3e-Lc13a (*takes you to* http://cks.nice.org.uk/diarrhoea-adults-assessment...)

tinyurl.com/CS3e-Lc13b (*takes you to* www.gov.uk/.../campylobacter-guidance-data-and-analysis)

Background information

- Take a travel history, as 50% of travellers returning from non-European destinations, particularly central America, South America and the Indian subcontinent, are likely to have a bacterial or parasitic cause for their diarrhoea.
- Blood in the stool may help in discriminating between non-self-limiting infectious and non-infective colitis. Around 40% of patients with *Campylobacter* infection have blood in their stool (compared with 10% of those whose infections are due to other causes), and bloody stools are also common in infection with toxogenic *E. coli*, *Salmonella*, *Shigella*, and *Yersinia*.
- Fever is present in around half of patients with infective diarrhoea, particularly in *Campylobacter* and rotavirus infections, compared with around 10% in non-infective diarrhoea.
- Headache seems to be most common in rotavirus infections, in which bloody stools are unusual, but it is a non-specific symptom and not a useful discriminator.
- C-reactive protein is more likely to be raised in gastroenteritis with a bacterial, rather than a viral, cause. It is of less value in diagnosing inflammatory bowel disease because its concentration is commonly below 10 mg/L in patients with ulcerative colitis but is raised in 75% of patients with Crohn's disease.
- High risk groups include older people and those with comorbidities, such as HIV infection and immunosuppression, who should be investigated at an early stage.

Long case 14 – Man with UTI

Brief to the doctor

Mr MN is a 24 year old man attending for the result of a urine test taken a week previously by your nurse practitioner.

Patient summary

Name	MN
Date of birth (Age)	24
Social and family history	Single Engineer
Past medical history	1 week ago – Nurse Practitioner Clinic: *"4/7 dysuria, frequency and urgency. Urine Prot tr, WBC +, Nit Pos. Send MSU. Trimethoprim 200mg bd 7/7. Pt will call me in 4d for result."*
Current medication	None
Investigations WBC RBC Scanty mixed growth	1 week ago MSU: $>10^7$/ml Nil ?significance

Tasks for the doctor

In this case, the tasks are to:
- review the patient's response to treatment and relate this to the MSU result
- answer the patient's questions about how he developed a UTI

Brief to the patient – more about the patient

1. Profile:

- MN, a 24 year old engineering graduate, has worked for an international mining company since graduating 2 years ago
- shares a rented flat with his girlfriend, a nurse at the local hospital; they plan to get married next year and buy their own flat
- enjoys an active lifestyle and likes to keep fit and healthy
- he developed urinary symptoms just over a week ago, attended the nurse practitioner's minor illness clinic and was told he probably had a UTI. He was given a prescription for antibiotics and told to phone the nurse back for the result

2. He is seeing the doctor today because:

- he has some questions he would like to discuss, rather than phone as instructed:
  - he is concerned about how he developed a UTI
  - his symptoms have not changed with the antibiotics – does this mean the nurse got the diagnosis or treatment wrong?
- the frequency and urgency symptoms are causing a lot of disruption and embarrassment – he usually works on sites around the country and keeps having to find toilets in a hurry

3. Additional information:

- If the doctor asks specifically:
  - his work mates have teased him that he might have an STD. He has not noticed any symptoms. He has not had sex with anyone other than his girlfriend for the past 6 months. If he has an STD, does this mean his girlfriend has been unfaithful? His girlfriend is on the Pill; they do not use condoms.
  - while working in South Africa 8 months ago, he had unprotected sex with a secretary working in his company's offices in Cape Town. This continued over a 2 month period until he returned to the UK. He feels very guilty about this and has not told his girlfriend about it. Before returning to the UK, he went to a GU Medicine Clinic and had tests, including HIV, and was told he was clear.
- He wants the doctor to explain:
  - how UTIs are 'caught'
  - the MSU result
  - why the antibiotics given by the nurse practitioner have not worked
  - what other diagnoses are possible
  - whether other tests or treatments are required

- He had an episode of discharge when he was a student, but was treated and checked afterwards and told he was clear.
- If the doctor talks about HIV, Mr MN will want to discuss:
  - why another test is required as he was told he was clear in South Africa
  - the implications on insurance and getting a mortgage
  - the implications for his girlfriend and any children they might have
  - how and where the test will be done – he is concerned that someone at the hospital will recognise his name as he and his girlfriend know and socialise with a lot of the staff there
  - if the test was positive, how would the practice deal with this? Would staff be told about his status? How would the practice guarantee confidentiality?
  - if the test was positive, what treatment would he have to have and what are the success rates nowadays?
  - given his job travelling round the country and sometimes abroad, are there any restrictions or precautions he would have to take?
- If the doctor talks about chlamydia, Mr MN will want to discuss:
  - how it is caught
  - if he has it, does this mean his girlfriend has been unfaithful?
  - could the South African clinic have missed it?
  - if he caught it in South Africa, why has it only just started giving him symptoms, and why has his girlfriend not had any symptoms?
  - will his girlfriend need to be tested and how should he raise this with her?
- Mr MN prefers simple straightforward honest answers to questions and will repeat questions to the doctor if he feels the doctor is evading answering or not giving unequivocal answers. He would rather be told all the possibilities, however bad, than be kept in the dark.

Approach to be taken

A. Data gathering, examination and clinical assessment skills

1. *Define the clinical problem: clarify why the patient has presented today*
   The doctor:
   - reads the patient information provided prior to the consultation
   - asks open questions to explore:
     - Mr MN's response to treatment – *"How are you getting on?"*
     - his concerns over why he has not improved – *"What do you make of that?"*
     - any other issues concerning him – *"Is there anything else you are worried this might be?"*
   - empathises with Mr MN over the practical effects of his symptoms
   - asks closed questions to clarify details about the symptoms, past history, and sexual history
   - obtains a sexual history in order to assesses Mr MN's risk of HIV or STDs

2. *Performs an appropriate physical or mental examination*
   - In this case, an examination is not required.

B. Clinical management skills

3. *Make an appropriate working diagnosis*
   - The doctor, based on the history and MSU result should suspect chlamydia.
   - This is a clinically sound hypothesis and is an appropriate use of probability.
   - The doctor integrates information to raise the possibility of HIV.

4. *Explain the problem to the patient using appropriate language*
   The doctor:
   - having quickly established that Mr MN is intelligent and eager to understand his symptoms, addresses his agenda
   - explains the MSU result and the possibility of chlamydia infection
   - provides information on chlamydia, in particular, how it may be asymptomatic for some time
   - explains that specific tests need to be done for chlamydia and that his girlfriend will need to be tested
   - should adopt a patient-centred approach to ensure he addresses the patient's concerns and expectations
   - uses chunking and checking information – *"Before I move on, can I check that I have got things clear?"*

5. *Provide holistic care and use resources effectively*
The doctor:
- practises evidence-based medicine – there is a likelihood of chlamydia given the MSU result, and a possibility of HIV given the history of unprotected sex in a high-risk country
- understands socioeconomic/cultural background – discusses ways of informing his girlfriend that she needs to be tested – *"Would you like to discuss how you might raise this matter with your girlfriend?"*
- is able to discuss the benefits and other implications of HIV testing – including insurance, mortgage, future health and travel
- provides Mr MN with verbal and written information on chlamydia and HIV

6. *Prescribe appropriately*
The doctor:
- advises Mr MN that a second HIV test is required before he can be told he is clear
- does not prescribe antibiotics as the diagnosis is not certain and other STDs must be excluded
- provides the patient with a referral letter to a GUM Clinic for investigation and consideration of HIV testing

7. *Specify the conditions and interval for follow-up*
The doctor:
- confirms understanding – *"Can I just check that I have explained things clearly – what is the plan for you?"*
- signposts Mr MN to information on chlamydia and HIV and to GUM Clinics where he could be tested
- offers a follow-up appointment to discuss any issues arising – safety netting

C. Interpersonal skills: know and treat this patient

8. *Achieve rapport*
The doctor:
- listens carefully to Mr MN's concerns about his symptoms not settling and the effects they have on him at work
- without embarrassment, sympathetically and sensitively elicits Mr MN's past sexual history
- places problem in psychosocial context – how it affects patient/girlfriend/ work
- understands his request for information on chlamydia
- displays empathy when raising the question of whether Mr MN is at risk of HIV and should have another test
- helps Mr MN explore ways of raising the issues with his girlfriend – *"Would you like to practise how you might tell her?"*

- answers Mr MN's questions using appropriate language
- is non-judgemental about Mr MN's past sexual experiences
- addresses the patient's specific concerns and expectations – *"Is there anything else you want to ask me?"*

9. *Give the patient the opportunity to be involved in significant management decisions*
   The doctor:
   - actively confirms the patient's understanding of the problem – *"Does this make sense to you?"*
   - shares thoughts/involves patient – *"If I were to say that having unprotected sex in South Africa may have exposed you to HIV, what would you say?"*
   - agrees balanced plans – *"Are you happy with this plan?"*

Debrief

This starts as a relatively straightforward clinical case; the real challenge is communication skills with the patient over the possibility of chlamydia, how he could have caught it and the implications on his relationship, and finally the issue of HIV. The ability to take a sexual history without being awkward or embarrassed is also tested.

Discuss how the doctor could, if needed, improve his performance. In particular, assess how the doctor:
- answered questions in language and style that satisfied Mr MN
- discussed the sensitive issues of infidelity, STDs and HIV
- developed empathy and trust
- managed time in the consultation – not wasting time gathering information at the expense of discussing the sensitive issues

Revising data gathering

What questions could the doctor ask to discover the patient's ideas, concerns, expectations and health beliefs?
- Ideas: "*You said that work colleagues have teased you about having an STD, could that be a possibility?*"
- Concerns: "*Would you like to discuss how chlamydia is caught and the range of symptoms it can cause?*"
- Expectations: "*The result of your urine test has not proven a normal infection; have you considered other possible causes?*"
- Health beliefs: "*You seem concerned that I am suggesting another HIV test even though you were given the 'all-clear' in South Africa, shall we talk about HIV testing?*"

Once the doctor has gathered sufficient information, how could he summarise the problem for the patient?
- Evaluate whether the doctor used appropriate language, paced his explanation, and whether the explanation was well organised and logical.

Relevant literature

BASHH (2014) *UK national guideline on the management of non-gonococcal urethritis*. British Association of Sexual Health and HIV. www.bashh.org

BASHH (2014) CEG 2014: *Guidance on tests for sexually transmitted infections*. British Association of Sexual Health and HIV. www.bashh.org

Background information

tinyurl.com/CS3e-Lc14a (*takes you to* www.fpa.org.uk/.../non-specific-urethritis)

If signs and symptoms of non-specific urethritis do occur, they usually show up within 2–4 weeks of contact with an infection, but they can sometimes appear within a day or two (depending on the cause of the inflammation). In mild cases, symptoms may not show up for several months. Signs and symptoms:

- A white or cloudy discharge from the tip of the penis, usually more noticeable first thing in the morning. Sometimes this discharge is seen only when massaged out of the penis.
- Difficulty, pain or a burning sensation when passing urine.
- The feeling of needing to pass urine frequently.
- Itching or irritation at the end of the urethra.

It is possible to be tested for signs of inflammation within a few days of having sex, but it may be necessary to wait up to two weeks before testing for infections such as chlamydia. Routine tests for *Mycoplasma genitalium* and *Ureaplasma urealyticum* are not currently widely available in the UK but may be offered at some clinics, particularly to men with persistent non-specific urethritis.

The tests may involve a doctor or nurse:

- using a swab to collect a sample of cells from the entrance of the urethra
- asking the patient to give a urine sample
- examining the penis.

A swab of urethral discharge and cells may be examined under the microscope straight away in GUM. Alternatively, urine tests may be used. Routine blood tests do not detect non-specific urethritis.

Long case 15 – Childhood bedwetting

Brief to the doctor

Mrs DJ is a 29 year old woman who presents (without her 6 year old son) asking for advice on his bedwetting.

Patient summary

Name	Tomas J
Date of birth (Age)	6
Social and Family History	One sister, age 3
Past medical history	Healthy – achieved appropriate milestones for age Seen occasionally for mild, seasonal URTIs
Repeat medication	None

Tasks for the doctor

In this case, the tasks are to:
- clarify the extent and nature of the bedwetting
- the effect of the bedwetting on Tomas and his family
- provide evidence-based advice on treatments

Brief to the patient – more about the patient

1. Profile:

- Mrs DJ is 29 year old housewife; her husband is a car mechanic
- both her children are healthy and developing as expected
- Mrs DJ is worried about her 6 year old son's bedwetting

2. She is seeing the doctor today because:

- she is concerned that Tomas still wets the bed at least 2 times per week. He has never been dry at night, but he is dry during the day. He has no medical problems and does not suffer from constipation or urine infections.
- he is a lovely child who is achieving well at school; he has lots of friends
- she has declined the sleep-overs to which Tomas has been invited as she thinks it would be embarrassing for him if he bed-wets on a sleepover – she worries about him being teased
- now that her daughter is 3, she would like to leave her children with her mum for a week so that she and her husband can go on holiday, but the frequent changing and washing of bedding creates a burden of housework and she feels guilty approaching her 56 year old mother
- nobody in the family has had a bedwetting problem
- she has tried restricting drinks for Tomas at night but this has not made much difference
- she thought the problem would resolve by age 5, but Tomas is now 6. Does he have a problem predisposing him to bedwetting? Should he be investigated? Does he need tablet treatments? Is there anything else she should do?

3. Additional information:

- if the doctor refers her to the health visitor, she would like to know what she should expect in terms of assessment and advice?
- if the doctor mentions different options to her, she expects to be advised on the efficacy of each before deciding on what she would like for Tomas

Approach to be taken

A. Data gathering, examination and clinical assessment skills

1. *Define the clinical problem: clarify why the patient has presented today*
   The doctor:
   - notes from the patient information provided that this is a 6 year old with no significant past medical history
   - asks mum open questions to explore the nature of the bedwetting (to make a diagnosis of primary nocturnal enuresis in a healthy, socially well adjusted 6 year old boy)
   - asks what has made her present today (to discover that Mrs DJ is thinking of leaving the children with her mum for a week in the school holidays to have a break with her husband)
   - asks closed questions to identify potentially reversible contributory factors: constipation, urinary tract infections, diet, stress (school problems / family discord / moving house), diabetes mellitus, ease of access to a toilet or potty, night lights, and bunk beds
   - excludes red flags: neurological problems, behaviour problems, sleep apnoea
   - elicits how the problem affects Tomas (embarrassment, social isolation, teasing by family members or friends)
   - elicits how the problem affects the family (parental anxiety / frustration / punishment / extra work of laundry / effect of interrupted sleep)
   - discovers her ideas that bedwetting should have ceased by age 6
   - discovers her concerns about the social restriction (sleep-overs / family holidays)
   - discovers her expectations for advice and a treatment plan

2. *Performs an appropriate physical or mental examination*
   - In this case, an examination is not required. However, make arrangements to examine Tomas (abdomen, genitalia, spine (tuft of hair/lipoma), knee jerks, and a dipstick urinalysis).

B. Clinical management skills

3. *Make an appropriate working diagnosis*
   - The doctor, based on the history, makes a working diagnosis of childhood primary nocturnal enuresis. There are no contributory factors.

4. *Explain the problem to the patient using appropriate language*
   The doctor:
   - contextualises the problem: 1 in 50 7 year olds wet the bed more than once a week and 15% get better without treatment each year. Children who are passing large volumes at night may not be producing sufficient

anti-diuretic hormone (ADH); small volumes may indicate small, irritable bladders; or the child may be sleeping so deeply that he is unaware of the sensation of a full bladder.

- having established the absence of red flags and contributory factors, provides general support and advice: signposting to ERIC (enuresis resource and information centre), using waterproof mattress coverings, avoiding caffeine after 3 pm, timing and amount of fluid intake
- refers to the health visitor for specific advice: star charts to reward getting out of bed to use the toilet, or enuresis alarms (bed or body-worn) for the child to learn to stop urinating when the alarm sounds – because they require the child's cooperation, alarms are usually reserved for children over 7 years
- advises Mrs DJ that drug treatment, with desmopressin, is appropriate for short periods such as sleep-overs or holidays away from home; desmopressin can be used in a 6 year old, and is effective while taken but bedwetting recurs on discontinuation

5. *Provide holistic care and use resources effectively*
   The doctor:
   - practises evidence-based medicine that is informed by national or local guidelines (www.nice.org.uk/guidance/qs70)
   - involves the health visitor in on-going treatment and support
   - does not refer to secondary care in the absence of red flags and contributory symptoms

6. *Prescribe appropriately*
   The doctor:
   - is aware of the indications and side-effects of desmopressin
   - discusses prescription but is unlikely to prescribe without having examined the child first; routine urinalysis is not required

7. *Specify the conditions and interval for follow-up*
   The doctor:
   - signposts Mrs DJ to information on nocturnal enuresis, such as www.eric.org.uk/
   - offers a follow-up appointment to examine Tomas

C. Interpersonal skills: know and treat this patient

8. *Achieve rapport*
   The doctor:
   - listens attentively to Mrs DJ's concerns regarding the continued bedwetting and its impact on the family
   - displays empathy to the workload and financial burden the bedwetting creates
   - addresses the patient's specific expectations about a long-term solution and what to do for sleep-overs and holidays
   - is sensitive in his queries regarding the parents' frustration and the possible punishment of the child

9. *Give the patient the opportunity to be involved in significant management decisions*
   The doctor:
   - shares his thoughts, for example, *"I am reassured by what you have told me about Tomas's physical and social development. I think this problem will resolve in time as his hormones and bladder mature. There are a few things we could do to help Tomas. I'll give you the options first and then you can tell me which you'd like to try."*
   - encourages autonomy and opinions – provides her with information so she feels able to choose the most appropriate option for Tomas and the family

Debrief

Discuss how the doctor could, if needed, improve his performance. In particular, assess whether the doctor:

- structured the history taking? For example, did the doctor preface his questions with *"I need to ask some questions to rule out serious illness – does Tomas have any of the following?"*
- assessed the impact of the bedwetting on the entire family? If so, how?
- addressed Mrs DJ's specific concerns? If so, how?
- made appropriate use of resources?
- outlined the reasons for follow-up?

If the consultation over-ran, did the doctor:

- ask open rather than closed questions when assessing contributory and red flag symptoms?
- provide overly detailed explanations of each option?
- signpost inadequately, that is, duplicate the services of the health visitor (or continence advisor) in providing detailed information and on-going support?

Revising data gathering

What questions could the doctor ask to discover the patient's ideas, concerns, expectations and health beliefs?

- Ideas: *"What is your understanding of bedwetting – causes, treatments and so on?"*
- Concerns: *"Is there anything in particular about the current situation that is worrying you?"*
- Expectations: *"When you came to see me today, was there anything in particular you'd hoped I'd do for you?"*
- Health beliefs: *"You seem concerned that your 6 year old hasn't achieved night-time dryness. Let's talk about this for a moment."*

Relevant literature

tinyurl.com/CS3e-Lc15a (*takes you to* https://pathways.nice.org.uk/pathways/bedwetting-nocturnal-enuresis-in-children-and-young-people)

Watson, L (2010) Enuresis. *InnovAiT*, **3**: 91–94.

Background information

Medical treatment is recommended from age 5, particularly if the child and family are motivated to engage in treatment.

Families often try simple behavioural therapies – such as fluid restriction, rewards, and taking the child to the toilet at night – as first attempts to manage the problem. More children became dry when rewarded and when lifted during the night. Avoid ineffective and even potentially harmful strategies, such as fluid restriction, retention control training (encouraging the child not to void for as long as possible to expand bladder capacity), and unnecessary drugs. Rewarding agreed behaviour (such as drinking adequately, voiding before sleep, and engaging in management) may be more effective than rewarding dry nights, which are out of the child's conscious control.

Enuresis alarms
Enuresis alarms are used in children over 7 years who are well motivated. Enuresis alarms can take several months to work and are usually needed for 3–5 months. They achieve a lower relapse rate than drug treatment, with 30–50% of children relapsing.

There are several types of alarm. They usually involve placement of a sensor in the child's underwear or in a pad underneath the child. The alarm sounds when it becomes wet. The alarm wakes the child who has to get out of bed to silence it. The child should then go to pass urine, dry off and help to remake his bed before going back to sleep. It is not necessary to reset the alarm that night. A baby monitor can be used to transmit the sound of the alarm to the parents' room. In time, the child learns to awaken before the alarm sounds or to sleep through the night without the need to pass urine. The treatment can be discontinued once a child has succeeded in being dry for 14 consecutive nights. An alarm can be used in conjunction with drug treatment if either therapy by itself is unsuccessful. Alarms are available from local enuresis clinics or from charities such as 'Education and Resources for Improving Childhood Continence' (ERIC).

Desmopressin is a synthetic analogue of antidiuretic hormone (ADH). It should not be given intranasally because of an increased incidence of side-effects. The usual oral dose is 200 mcg taken at bedtime in children over 5 years (preferably over 7 years). Limit fluid intake to a minimum from 1 hour before dose until 8 hours afterwards. Do not continue for longer than 3 months; stop for 1 week for reassessment. Stop taking desmopressin during an episode of vomiting and diarrhoea (until fluid balance is normal).

Long case 16 - Prostate cancer

Brief to the doctor

Mr OP is a 74 year old man who saw a locum 4 days ago because of urinary symptoms. The locum arranged tests for MSU, FBC, U&Es, LFTs and PSA. Mr OP attends today for the results.

Patient summary

Name	OP
Date of birth (Age)	74
Social and family history	Married Retired carpenter and joiner No FH CVD
Past medical history	4 days ago – Locum: *"Frequency, nocturia ×4, dribbling. Urine NAD. Abdo NAD. RE hard nodular left lobe prostate. Check bloods and review prior to referral. Pt not told prostate feels suspicious."*
Current medication	None

Investigations

4 days ago:

Hb	11.2 g/dl (12–15)
MCV	78.4 (83–105)
WBC	2.3 (4–11)
ESR	84
Na	130 (135–145)
K	3.4 (3.5–5)
Urea	5.6 (2.5–6.7)
Creatinine	76 (70–150)
AlkP	185 (95–280)
AST	28
ALT	31 (10–45)
PSA	10 (<4.0)

Tasks for the doctor

In this case, the tasks are to:
- review results and the locum's clinical findings
- explain the results and the necessary actions to the patient
- deal with the patient's anxiety over the possible diagnosis

Brief to the patient – more about the patient

1. Profile:

- Mr OP is a 74 year old retired carpenter and joiner
- he likes to keeps active, although after a hip replacement 4 years ago he has not been as active as he hoped he would be
- he has been troubled with hesitancy, weak stream, spraying, straining, intermittency, incomplete emptying and terminal dribbling for the past year, but things have got worse over the past 2 months
- he feels well in himself, but gets tired easily – he attributes this to his age
- he does not like to make a fuss and believes doctors should not be questioned – they are experts and he should take their advice

2. He is seeing the doctor today because:

- the locum doctor took some tests and told him to come back to see one of the regular doctors for the results
- a lot of his friends have prostate problems and are taking tablets that help; he expects the doctor is going to start him on these today

3. Additional information:

- If the doctor asks specifically:
  - symptoms – difficulty starting to pee, taking longer to empty his bladder, straining to empty, the stream sprays, stream is weak and dribbles at the end; he has not seen blood in the urine
  - he has not lost any weight and has no other symptoms
  - his father's brother died of prostate cancer. His father died of old age. His uncle was treated by orchidectomy – Mr OP is horrified at this treatment.
- If the doctor suggests that the results are suspicious or that referral for more tests is required, Mr OP will ask if there is a possibility of cancer.
- He is still sexually active.
- His wife had a small heart attack 2 years ago, but is well and active now. He tries not to trouble her with things because she is a worrier and he is concerned that worrying will strain her heart.
- He has two children who both live locally and visit regularly.
- He has not considered the possibility of having cancer because he feels well, unlike his uncle who was ill and lost a lot of weight.
- If the doctor mentions cancer:
  - he will get very anxious about his wife, possible treatments and prognosis
  - he will want the doctor to explain what treatments are possible and their success
  - he will want to discuss what he should tell his wife and whether it will affect her heart

Approach to be taken

A. Data gathering, examination and clinical assessment skills

1. *Define the clinical problem: clarify why the patient has presented today*
   The doctor:
   - reads the patient information provided prior to the consultation
   - asks open questions to explore what the locum told Mr OP and what Mr OP suspects might be the cause of his symptoms: "*Can you tell me what the locum said to you?*" and "*What do you think might be the cause?*"
   - asks closed questions to clarify Mr OP's symptoms and family history
   - responds to non-verbal cues: "*You look like you weren't expecting to be told you needed to be referred, am I right?*"

2. *Performs an appropriate physical or mental examination*
   - In this case, an examination is not required.

B. Clinical management skills

3. *Make an appropriate working diagnosis*
   - The doctor integrates information from the history, the locum's examination and blood results and makes a working diagnosis of suspected prostatic cancer.

4. *Explain the problem to the patient using appropriate language*
   The doctor:
   - informs Mr OP that the blood test results and the locum's examination are not normal and that further tests at the hospital are indicated
   - uses a patient-centred approach to address Mr OP's concerns and expectations – "*I cannot say whether this is cancer or not until you have had some tests at the hospital*"
   - checks the patient's understanding: "*This has been a bit of a shock for you, can I just go over what we have just talked about before moving on to the next bit?*"
   - provides some information on what tests may be required, and what treatments are available: transrectal ultrasound, biopsy, bone scans, treatments depend on stage and assessed risk and range from active surveillance only through surgery to radiotherapy and chemo- and hormone therapy

5. *Provide holistic care and use resources effectively*
   The doctor:
   - practises evidence-based medicine and is informed by national or local guidelines – NICE (2008) *Prostate cancer: diagnosis and treatment*

- allows Mr OP time to explore his anxieties about telling his wife his possible diagnosis
- provides Mr OP with information if required

6. *Prescribe appropriately*
The doctor:
- is aware of national and local guidelines:
  ○ for suspected cancer referrals: NICE (2015) *Suspected cancer: recognition and referral* (NG12 – www.nice.org.uk/guidance/ng12)
  ○ for prostate cancer: NICE (2014) *Prostate cancer: diagnosis and treatment* (CG175 – www.nice.org.uk/guidance/cg175)

7. *Specify the conditions and interval for follow-up*
The doctor:
- offers a follow-up appointment to discuss any issues arising from his outpatient attendance or if Mr OP has any questions or concerns
- safety netting – "*You should have received an appointment to be seen within the next 2 weeks; let me know if you have heard nothing in one week's time*"
- arranges to see Mr OP after the hospital appointment

C. Interpersonal skills: know and treat this patient

8. *Achieve rapport*
The doctor:
- sensitively informs Mr OP about the need for referral
- explores and clarifies Mr OP's concerns and expectations: "*You look concerned. Is there anything particular worrying you?*"
- listens attentively to Mr OP's concerns about his wife
- displays empathy: "*I understand why you are worried about the effect this might have on your wife; would you like to discuss this for a while?*"

9. *Give the patient the opportunity to be involved in significant management decisions*
The doctor:
- actively confirms the patient's understanding of the problem: "*What does all this mean to you?*"
- provides the patient with information by answering his questions, but does not raise unnecessary alarm as the diagnosis has not been confirmed
- supports the patient by discussing his concerns about possible treatments (particularly orchidectomy) and how to tell his wife

Debrief

This case focuses on the doctor's ability to raise the possibility of bad news.

Discuss how the doctor could, if needed, improve his performance. In particular, assess how the doctor:
- managed time in the consultation – did s/he spend too much time reviewing symptoms and not enough on answering Mr OP's concerns?
- raised the need for further tests and answered Mr OP's question about whether or not he had cancer

Revising data gathering

What questions could the doctor ask to discover the patient's ideas, concerns, expectations and health beliefs?
- Ideas: "*I understand that you wouldn't want the same treatment your uncle had; do you know anything about other treatments?*"
- Concerns: "*I understand that cancer is a frightening word, would you like to discuss prostate cancer in more detail?*"
- Expectations: "*I am going to refer you to the hospital; would you like me to outline what tests they are likely to want to do?*"
- Health beliefs: "*You are worried that this might affect your wife's health; would you like to spend some time talking about this?*"

Relevant literature

Cancer Research UK: www.cancerresearchuk.org/about-cancer/prostate-cancer

A framework for breaking bad news: www.skillscascade.com/badnews.htm

Background information

If a patient presents with

- Inflammatory or obstructive LUTS
- Erectile dysfunction
- Haematuria
- Lower back pain
- Bone pain
- Weight loss, especially in the elderly

screen for UTI first, and if absent, do a PSA, then a digital rectal examination (DRE).

The serum PSA level alone should not lead to biopsy.

The man and his partner should be given adequate time and information to make the decision. The information should include the risks and benefits of biopsy.

If the patient is obviously high risk – for example, high PSA and evidence of bone metastases on investigation – biopsy is unnecessary.

Long case 17 – Painful calf

Brief to the doctor

Mrs RD is a 29 year old woman who presents with a painful left calf.

Patient summary

Name	RD
Date of birth (Age)	29
Social and Family History	Married, no children Teacher Non-smoker
Past medical history	Difficulty sleeping (1 year ago) – given zopiclone Cervical smear 5 years ago – normal
Repeat medication	None

Tests	Values are from 6 months ago
BMI	24.2
BP	118/72
	Value from 1 year ago
PHQ score	6/27

Tasks for the doctor

In this case, the tasks are to:
- clarify whether Mrs RD's fears about having a DVT are well-founded
- negotiate appropriate and timely investigation
- explain the nature of the investigation(s) in simple, jargon-free language

Brief to the patient – more about the patient

1. Profile:

- Mrs RD is a 29 year old woman who works as a teacher in the local primary school
- when she married 4 months ago, she stopped taking the combined oral contraceptive pill (Microgynon) which she had used, without problems, since the age of 19; she hopes to get pregnant and her period is 2 days late – she has not done a pregnancy test as yet

2. She is seeing the doctor today because:

- her left calf has been painful for 36 hours – it feels swollen and warm to the touch
- she drove down from Edinburgh to London 3 days ago; there were problems on the road and the journey took 11 hours, but there was no opportunity during the 3 hour delay to leave the car
- she does not have a past history of deep vein thrombosis (DVT), is no longer on Microgynon, and has not had recent surgery. Her sister (aged 28) had a DVT during the 20th week of her pregnancy. Nobody else in the family has had a DVT or pulmonary embolus (PE).
- she has not done any recent strenuous physical exercise, nor does she feel unwell in herself

3. Additional information:

- Mrs RD is worried that she may be pregnant and she may have a DVT
- she expects a referral to the hospital for a scan
- her sister was given injections to treat the DVT – will she be put on injections too? She has needle-phobia and does not believe that she will manage to self-inject.

Approach to be taken

A. Data gathering, examination and clinical assessment skills

1. *Define the clinical problem: clarify why the patient has presented today*
   The doctor:
   - reads the patient information provided prior to the consultation
   - asks open questions to explore the nature and duration of the symptoms
   - empathises with Mrs RD's concerns that this may be a DVT
   - asks closed questions to assess whether the patient is at high risk for DVT: previous history of DVT, recent surgery, recent immobility, malignancy?
   - asks about PE symptoms: shortness or breath, pleuritic chest pain, haemoptysis?
   - works through the diagnostic sieve to rule out other possible causes of a painful calf, such as cellulitis, lymphangitis, muscle strain, a ruptured Baker's cyst, or venous insufficiency. The doctor could sign-post his systematic questioning of the differential diagnosis by prefacing his questions with: *"I need to ask some questions to rule out all the possible causes of a sore calf – do you have any of the following symptoms: a red rash on the calf, feeling unwell in yourself, muscle strain from sport or an injury?"*.
   - asks about the possibility of pregnancy, an important red flag
   - discovers Mrs RD's idea that she has a DVT, her concern that she will need to treat the DVT by self injecting, her expectation of a referral to hospital for a scan and her belief that DVTs are treated by subcutaneous heparin

2. *Performs an appropriate physical or mental examination*
   - An examination is required and should be guided by the Wells scoring system – see tinyurl.com/CS3e-Lc17a (*takes you to* www.nice.org.uk/guidance/cg144/...)
   - Look for:
     - tenderness along entire deep vein system
     - swelling of entire leg
     - measure the calf circumference 10 cm below the tibial tuberosity and look for >3 cm difference in calf circumference
     - pitting oedema confined to the symptomatic leg
     - collateral dilated superficial veins (non-varicose)
     - the absence of signs pointing to an alternative diagnosis, such as cellulitis, congestive cardiac failure, muscle sprains or a Baker's cyst
   - In this patient, assume the only sign present is moderate tenderness (4/10) in the posterior aspect of the left calf which is worse when the patient stands up or when you passively dorsiflex her ankle.

B. Clinical management skills

3. *Make an appropriate working diagnosis*
   - The doctor, based on the history and examination, makes a working diagnosis of DVT. If the patient is not pregnant, the risk is low and a D-dimer test should be done. If the patient is pregnant, the risk is moderate to high and an ultrasound scan should be organised.

4. *Explain the problem to the patient using appropriate language*
   The doctor:
   - having clarified that Mrs RD has a good idea of what a DVT is based on her sister's experience, addresses her agenda
   - explains that further investigation (blood test or ultrasound scan) depends on whether or not she is pregnant – the doctor organises a pregnancy test
   - addresses her idea that she has a DVT. She may have a DVT, but further investigation is needed before a diagnosis can be made. Only 50% of patients with classic signs of a DVT actually have one.
   - Addresses her concerns: she is worried about self-injecting subcutaneous heparin. If she is pregnant and has a DVT (two assumptions at present), subcutaneous heparin is needed. If she is not pregnant and has a DVT, a brief period of subcutaneous injection is followed by oral warfarin therapy. The fact that injections are subcutaneous (rather than intramuscular) and may only be needed for a brief period may be reassuring to the patient.
   - Addresses her expectations: a scan is needed only if her pregnancy test is positive, or if her D-dimer result is positive.

5. *Provide holistic care and use resources effectively*
   The doctor:
   - practises evidence-based medicine
   - is informed by national or local guidelines: tinyurl.com/CS3e-Lc17b (*takes you to* https://cks.nice.org.uk/deep-vein-thrombosis#!scenario)

6. *Prescribe appropriately*
   The doctor:
   - is aware of national and local guidelines
   - does not prescribe until further information is available

7. *Specify the conditions and interval for follow-up*
   The doctor:
   - arranges for a pregnancy test. If positive, arranges for a scan. If negative, arranges for a D-dimer test.
   - if DVT is suspected on clinical grounds, further assessment and definitive diagnosis on the day of presentation is ideal

C. Interpersonal skills: know and treat this patient

8. *Achieve rapport*
   The doctor:
   - listens attentively to Mrs RD's concerns about having a DVT
   - understands her request for an ultrasound scan and deals with the request appropriately and with sensitivity
   - gently challenges or corrects the patient's assumption that she has a DVT requiring treatment with subcutaneous heparin

9. *Give the patient the opportunity to be involved in significant management decisions*
   The doctor:
   - negotiates with the patient when the pregnancy test will be done
   - gives the patient sufficient information to appreciate that time is of the essence and definitive testing should be completed within 24 hours of presentation

Debrief

Discuss how the doctor could, if needed, improve his performance. In particular, assess whether the doctor:
- took a systematic history, quickly eliciting the risk factors for DVT, and working through the diagnostic sieve
- discussed and prioritised the order of the investigations, while addressing the patient's expectation of a scan appropriately
- explained the investigations (D-dimer testing) in simple language

If the consultation over-ran, was the doctor:
- systematic in his history taking – were questions asked without appropriate signposting?
- systematic, thorough and confident in his examination technique?
- logical and organised in arranging further investigation and follow-up?

Revising data gathering

What questions could the doctor ask to discover the patient's ideas, concerns, expectations and health beliefs?
- Ideas: *"What do you imagine the treatment for DVT will be?"*
- Concerns: *"With regard to DVTs, what are you most worried about?"*
- Expectations: *"How was your sister's DVT diagnosed? Did you also expect to be scanned?"*
- Health beliefs: *"You have good grounds for suspecting a DVT. Let's just talk about how we go about confirming or disproving a DVT."*

Relevant literature

tinyurl.com/CS3e-Lc17b (*takes you to* https://cks.nice.org.uk/deep-vein-thrombosis#!scenario)

www.youtube.com/watch?v=Y2XHP-aaDpc – presentation on DVT by Stephen Bright

tinyurl.com/CS3e-Lc17c (*takes you to* www.nice.org.uk/guidance/cg144/chapter/recommendations)

Background information

The Wells score is the most widely validated method used to assess a patient's risk of current DVT. A Wells score of less than 2 means that the patient has a low risk of DVT, while those with a score of 2 or more are at high risk of current DVT.

A D-dimer test demonstrates the presence of blood clot degradation products. With a negative predictive value of 97.7%, it is a useful test for ruling out DVT.

A negative D-dimer blood test and a Wells score of less than 2 are effective in ruling out a DVT without the need for duplex ultrasound.

If DVT is left untreated about 50% of patients will develop a symptomatic pulmonary embolism, which carries a 10% risk of death within one hour of onset of initial symptoms. The main goal of treatment is to prevent pulmonary embolism, propagation of the clot, and recurrence of the DVT.

Standard treatment for DVT is immediate anticoagulation with subcutaneous low molecular weight heparins for at least five days, and that the patient should simultaneously take oral anticoagulants such as warfarin for at least three months. The duration of oral treatment depends on the cause of the DVT and whether it can be eliminated or not. Anticoagulation (without compression stockings) decreases the risk of pulmonary embolism to 3.8%, the risk of recurrent DVT to 30%, and the risk of post-thrombotic syndrome to 82%.

Long case 18 – Leg ulcer

Brief to the doctor

Miss QR is an 85 year old lady who is usually seen regularly in surgery by your senior partner (Dr Smith). She has requested a home visit because she has knocked her leg and it is 'leaking water'.

Patient summary

Name	QR
Date of birth (Age)	85
Social and family history	Lives alone in privately owned old people's flat Warden on site
Past medical history	Hypertension – 30 years Leg oedema – 4 years Osteoarthritis both knees – 15 years Obesity – 45 years
	Saw Dr Smith 1 month ago: "*No great change. BP 140/84, oedema to just above knees. Walking with a stick. Blood test done. No change in medication.*"
Current medication	Lisinopril 20 mg daily Furosemide 40 mg twice daily
Investigations	1 month ago – FBC, U&Es and fasting glucose all normal

Tasks for the doctor

In this case, the tasks are to:
- explore and clarify Miss QR's concerns
- formulate an appropriate clinical and social management plan, utilising other members of the PCT

Brief to the patient – more about the patient

1. Profile:

- Miss QR is an 85 year old lady who lives alone in a privately owned old flat in an old people's block with a resident warden
- she has long-standing hypertension and osteoarthritis in her knees. She has been overweight most of her life and knows she should lose weight, but has no motivation to do so. For the past 4 years her legs have been swollen and this is limiting her mobility significantly.
- she attends surgery every 3 months for a check with Dr Smith
- she has no family history of CVD or DM

2. She is seeing the doctor today because:

- she knocked her leg on the corner of a coffee table last week, causing a superficial wound which she put a plaster on initially, but she started to leak fluid from the wound and when she removed the plaster she tore off skin, leaving a superficial raw area
- the leg has continued to leak. Friends have bought dressings and bandages from the local chemist who has now suggested to them that she should be seen. She has to sit with plastic bags under her leg to prevent the carpet getting soiled and has had to put a waterproof mattress cover on her bed. She is very meticulous about hygiene and finds the leaking fluid repugnant.
- she is terrified of developing leg ulcers
- she is very proud that her blood tests for kidney function, diabetes and cholesterol have always been normal and feels that this justifies her belief that there would be no real benefit to her if she lost weight
- she feels well despite the current problem

3. Additional information:

- If the doctor asks specifically:
  - she lives on the first floor, but there is a lift
  - she has been elevating her legs on a low stool
- She will not accept hospital admission unless she is very ill.
- She has a home help who visits once weekly to clean and do her shopping. Miss QR can cook for herself and is completely independent.
- She believes a District Nurse should be asked to visit and dress her leg.
- She is struggling to cope with her single stick and believes a frame might be a better option; she is reluctant to ask for this as she feels she is being over-demanding when resources in the NHS are scarce.
- If the doctor examines her:

System	Examination findings
General	No pallor. Grossly overweight.
CVS	HR 76 SR. HS 1+2 +nil. BP 136/82 Lungs clear Pitting oedema to mid-thigh level Unable to palpate pedal pulses due to oedema
Abdo	No mass. No organomegaly. No ascites.
Legs	Oedema as noted OA knees with valgus deformity on right 4 × 4cm superficial ulcer left shin. Very thin shiny surrounding skin with some small scattered vesicles. No surrounding cellulitis and no slough on ulcer. No evidence of infection. Serous fluid leaking from ulcer.

Approach to be taken

A. Data gathering, examination and clinical assessment skills

1. *Define the clinical problem: clarify why the patient has presented today*
   The doctor:
   - reads the patient information provided prior to the consultation
   - asks open questions to explore why she has asked for a home visit a week after injuring her leg – *"Have you any thoughts about what can be done to help you?"*
   - empathises with her about the leaking fluid
   - asks closed questions to clarify details about her past history and current medication, and her general health at present

2. *Performs an appropriate physical or mental examination*
   - Explains that an examination is required using appropriate language.
   - Performs a targeted examination to assess wound and degree of heart failure – this should include looking at the wound, assessing the extent of her oedema, checking JVP and listening to her heart and lungs.
   - Examination addresses patient's concerns – to see whether she has an ulcer.

B. Clinical management skills

3. *Make an appropriate working diagnosis*
   - The doctor, based on the history and examination, makes a working diagnosis of leg ulcer in a lady with heart failure.

4. *Explain the problem to the patient using appropriate language*
   The doctor:
   - explains why the ulcer has developed and why it has continued to leak fluid
   - addresses the patient's concerns and expectations – *"There is a good chance we can get the ulcer to heal as it is shallow, but we will need to decrease your leg swelling to help this happen."*

5. *Provide holistic care and use resources effectively*
   The doctor:
   - arranges for the District Nurse to visit to assess the ulcer and provide appropriate dressings and monitor response
   - explains what the District Nurse is likely to do – Doppler Ankle Brachial Pressure Index (ABPI)
   - provides some information on what Miss QR can do to help herself – good skin care, low salt intake, importance of mobility and exercise, leg elevation when immobile
   - identifies the social (decreased mobility) and psychological (finds the leaking fluid repugnant) impact of this diagnosis on Miss QR

- uses PCT and other resources – District Nurse and physiotherapy/OT assessment of whether a frame might enable safer mobility than her current stick

6. *Prescribe appropriately*
The doctor:
- decides to see if rest and elevation will be beneficial before altering treatment
- decides to await the result of the ABPI before formulating an ulcer management plan: compression bandaging with or without pentoxifylline, which is believed to increase microcirculatory blood flow

7. *Specify the conditions and interval for follow-up*
The doctor:
- offers a follow-up appointment either with him/herself or with Dr Smith to monitor progress
- confirms understanding – *"Is there anything I haven't explained or you don't understand?"*

C. Interpersonal skills: know and treat this patient

8. *Achieve rapport*
The doctor:
- explores and clarifies Miss QR's concerns – *"Is there anything in particular you are worried about?"*
- places problem in psychosocial context – *"How are you coping with all this on your own?"*
- supports the long relationship Miss QR has with Dr Smith
- addresses the patient's specific concerns and expectations – District Nurse visit and provision of a frame

9. *Give the patient the opportunity to be involved in significant management decisions*
The doctor:
- actively confirms patient's understanding of the problem – *"Have I adequately explained to you why your leg is leaking fluid?"*
- uses time as a therapeutic tool – no medication change, monitor effects of ulcer treatment and elevation
- encourages autonomy and opinions – *"Have you had any thoughts on what I can do to help?"*
- supports and congratulates her in looking after the ulcer initially and preventing infection

Debrief

Discuss how the doctor could, if needed, improve his performance. In particular, assess how the doctor:
- established rapport with a patient who usually saw another doctor
- explored Miss QR's concerns and beliefs
- explained the possible management plans that may result from the ABPI results

Revising data gathering

What questions could the doctor ask to discover the patient's ideas, concerns, expectations and health beliefs?
- Ideas: "*Why do you think the wound has not healed as quickly as you expected?*"
- Concerns: "*Is there anything you are particularly worried about?*"
- Expectations: "*You have done really well to keep the wound clean, but it isn't healing as you expected. What do you think needs to be done now?*"
- Health beliefs: "*The pharmacist advised getting the wound checked – let's discuss wound healing briefly.*"

Relevant literature

SIGN (2010) *Management of chronic venous leg ulcers*. Clinical guideline No. 120. tinyurl.com/CS3e-Lc18a (*takes you to* www.sign.ac.uk/guidelines/...)

Simon DA, Dix FP and McCollum CN (2004) Management of venous leg ulcers. *BMJ*, **328**(7452): 1358–62.

Background information

Examine for location, size, colour and degree of necrosis, and palpate the peripheral arterial pulses. Check for complications, such as osteomyelitis and the development of squamous cell carcinoma in the base of the ulcer.

If peripheral arterial pulses are absent, investigation of the ankle-brachial index using Doppler ultrasound will help discriminate venous disease from arterial disease.

Treatment of venous ulcers is either conservative (bed rest, leg elevation, local treatment and compression) or surgical (such as superficial and perforating vein ablation and deep vein reconstruction).

Resources for patients

In USA: www.veinforum.org/patients.html

In New Zealand: tinyurl.com/CS3e-Lc18b (*takes you to* http://www.vascular.co.nz/chronic_venous_insufficiency%20and%20leg%20ulceration.htm)

Long case 19 – A list of symptoms

Brief to the doctor

Mrs SW is a 52 year old woman who presents with a list of problems:
1. pain in right calf
2. voice is hoarse
3. I had recent blood tests – what are the results?
4. I think I'm going through the menopause – feeling low, tired, no sex drive, weight gain

Patient summary

Name	SW
Date of birth (Age)	52
Social and Family History	Married for 28 years with one child (27)
	Works from home providing IT support
Past medical history	Sleep disorders (8 months ago) – issued zopiclone
	Right leg sciatica (8 months ago) – issued analgesia
	Voice hoarseness (3 years ago) – no abnormalities found by ENT; assumed related to gastric reflux
	Intermittent asthma (from teenager)
Repeat medication	Diprobase 500 g as directed (AD)
	Seretide 125 evohaler Cfc-free 100 µg / puff (AD)
	Ventolin evohaler Cfc-free 100 µg / puff (AD)
	Lansoprazole 30 mg once daily × 28

Consultation note by Dr Brown (4 weeks ago):
'Voice hoarseness: has had previous episodes and investigations by ENT in the past. No evidence of cancer and felt related to gastric reflux. Gargles after using steroid inhalers. Has been having more reflux symptoms lately despite cutting down alcohol dramatically from 50 units per week and changing diet. Last week, only had 4 glasses of wine in total. O/E: no cervical lymph nodes felt. Throat OK. Chest clear. No creps or wheeze. Plan: Trial of doubling PPI. Get bloods for general health screen. Review thereafter.'

Blood tests	Tests were done two weeks ago
Hb	12.5 g/dl (12–15)
MCV	102 (83–105)
Liver functions tests	normal
Renal function	normal
TSH	4.32 (0.35–5.5)
Fasting glucose	6.2 (3–5.5)
Total cholesterol	5.7
HDL	1.1
H. pylori	negative

Tasks for the doctor

In this case, the tasks are to:

- negotiate the problem list, prioritising appropriately
- discuss the blood results, especially the abnormal fasting glucose
- discuss the menopausal symptoms
- establish that the calf pain and hoarse voice are long-standing problems, without recent red-flags, and agree review of these issues at follow-up appointments

Brief to the patient – more about the patient

1. Profile:

- Mrs SW is a 52 year old woman who has worked from home for the last 6 months. She misses the social interaction of working in an office environment and now feels lonely and low.
- she is happily married; her husband has noticed the increased alcohol consumption, which she has attributed to helping her sleep at night
- Mrs SW doesn't see the doctor often and because she is worried about her health, she presents with a list of symptoms. The list also helps her to remember what she wants to discuss. She is getting forgetful these days, a sign of the menopause, she thinks.

2. She is seeing the doctor today because:

- she has had an intermittent dull pain (3/10) in her right calf, worse on standing up from gardening, since her sciatica 8 months ago. The pain does not interrupt sleep, but is an irritating niggle that rarely interferes with everyday activities. She wants to know if she should continue with the exercises the physiotherapist gave her, or whether she needs to see the physiotherapist again for further assessment and treatment.
- she still has an intermittent hoarse voice, but things are much better. Dr Brown spoke to her about reducing her alcohol intake and taking lansoprazole 30 mg for 1 month. This has helped but she has run out of tablets. A repeat script is required but she doesn't know if she should take 15 mg or 30 mg of lansoprazole now.
- she had blood tests done. Dr Brown wanted to check that she was not anaemic or diabetic or had thyroid problems, possible causes of her tiredness. She does not believe she has these conditions. Dr Brown wanted the other tests as 'a general health screen in the over 40s'. When told about the raised fasting glucose, she is adamant that she had fasted, and she is surprised and slightly worried by the result: what does it mean, and what does she need to do about it? She does not have symptoms of DM. No one in her family has DM.
- she is worried about her menopausal symptoms: feeling low, tired, no sex drive, weight gain and irregular periods for the last 4 months. Flushing occurs, but infrequently, so this is not a major issue. Mrs SW feels she lacks the energy to exercise, socialize, and make more friends. If she socialized more, she'd not drink at home during the evening. She wants to get her energy back.
- she attributes her lack of energy to the menopause – her 'idea'
- she is concerned about getting a DVT from HRT seeing that she already has a 'weak calf'

- she expects to be told about the pros and cons of HRT; she does not expect a prescription for HRT today, but she does expect a prescription for lansoprazole

3. Additional information:

- if the doctor offers her a prescription for HRT, she says she'd like to read up on it first. She'd also like to consider alternatives such as St John's Wort or valerian for sleep. She expects the doctor to signpost her to suitable information.

Approach to be taken

A. Data gathering, examination and clinical assessment skills

1. *Define the clinical problem: clarify why the patient has presented today*
   The doctor:
   - makes use of the existing patient information provided prior to the consultation
   - empathises with Mrs SW's comments about needing to make a list because of her 'poor memory'
   - asks the patient to read out the whole list to gauge which problems need urgent attention, which can be dealt with quickly, and which may need attention at a later date. One way of dealing with the list may be to respond with *"OK, that sounds like a reasonable list, all of which need attention. I also need to talk to you about your blood results. Shall we start with that and see how we get on in our ten minutes. If it's OK with you, we'll also make a plan for dealing with those things we may not have time for today."*
   - asks questions to explore how reliable the fasting blood glucose result is and makes arrangements for a second fasting glucose or HbA1c blood test
   - asks open questions to explore what Mrs SW means by menopausal symptoms, which symptoms have the greatest adverse impact on her life and what her expectations of treatment are, thereby eliciting the story of lacking energy and the expectation of treatment to restore her drive
   - asks closed questions to clarify details about her periods, and possible contra-indications to HRT
   - asks about red flags for calf pain (recent swelling or pain, recent long periods of immobility), and hoarse voice (particularly hoarseness that deteriorated over the past month despite proton pump inhibitors)
   - discovers Mrs SW's idea that her lack of energy is due to the menopause, her concern about the risk of DVT with HRT, and her expectation for further information about HRT and a prescription for a lansoprazole

2. *Performs an appropriate physical or mental examination*
   - In this case, an examination is not required.

B. Clinical management skills

3. *Make an appropriate working diagnosis*
   The doctor, based on the history, makes a working diagnosis of:
   - possible disorders of glucose metabolism requiring further investigation (HbA1c)
   - peri-menopausal symptoms

4. *Explain the problem to the patient using appropriate language*
The doctor:
- explains that a diagnosis should not be made from a single blood test – the doctor organises an HbA1c and appropriately refers to the phlebotomist
- provides information on the treatment of peri-menopausal symptoms: indicates that HRT may increase energy levels, SSRIs may help with flushing and valerian may help sleep; St John's wort is an enzyme inducer and may interfere with prescribed medication
- explains the risks and benefits of HRT in appropriate language, and addresses the patient's particular concern regarding the risk of DVT on HRT
- checks the patient's understanding at each point – if understanding is good, the doctor moves forward to the next item on the patient's list
- prescribes an appropriate dose of lansoprazole for one month and negotiates review
- negotiates review of the calf pain, explaining that a thorough reassessment of the sciatica and calf pain is required prior to making a decision regarding referral to physiotherapy. Alternatively, if the physiotherapy department had offered the patient an open-access appointment on discharge, she could call them directly for advice.

5. *Provide holistic care and use resources effectively*
The doctor:
- prioritises the issues effectively
- makes balanced plans which are either doctor- or patient-centred as appropriate; for example, dealing with the raised fasting glucose is doctor-centred and dealing with the peri-menopausal symptoms is patient-centred
- discusses conventional and complementary medicines, if Mrs SW is interested in the latter, for the treatment of her peri-menopausal symptoms; advice follows national or local guidelines (http://cks.library.nhs.uk/menopause)

6. *Prescribe appropriately*
The doctor:
- is aware of national and local guidelines: tinyurl.com/CS3e-Lc19a (*takes you to* https://cks.nice.org.uk/dyspepsia-unidentified-cause)
- checks the patient's understanding of the medication and the amounts of medication required

7. *Specify the conditions and interval for follow-up*
The doctor:
- signposts Mrs SW to information on the menopause
- offers a follow-up appointment to discuss issues not dealt with today; in particular, review of the voice hoarseness / GORD and calf pain / sciatica is arranged

C. Interpersonal skills: know and treat this patient

8. *Achieve rapport*
The doctor:
- listens attentively to Mrs SW's recitation of her list without interruption, acknowledging that concern for her ability to remember everything prompted its writing
- understands her request for information on HRT, a repeat script for a PPI and review of her sciatica; the doctor is sympathetic and outlines his intention to address these issues today and at future appointments
- displays empathy to her lack of energy and supports her in her attempt to change her lifestyle
- is non-judgemental about the patient's alcohol intake and congratulates her on the reduction she's made
- addresses the patient's specific concerns and expectations

9. *Give the patient the opportunity to be involved in significant management decisions*
The doctor:
- encourages autonomy and opinions – provides Mrs SW with a brief outline on treatment options and signposts to appropriate resources on HRT management
- suggests further appointments with appropriate members of the PCT for future review

Debrief

Discuss how the doctor could, if needed, improve his performance. In particular, assess whether the doctor:
- negotiated the patient's list? Was this done in a sensitive manner?
- established and maintained rapport? If so, how?
- addressed Mrs SW's specific expectations? If so, how?
- discussed and signposted to appropriate HRT, including CAM?
- safety netted? If so, how?

If the consultation over-ran, did the doctor:
- spend too much time negotiating the list?
- ask too many questions about all the presenting issues before deciding on the ones to tackle?
- provide detailed information when outlining the main points would have sufficed? Remember that if the actor–patient is unhappy with the amount and detail of information provided, they are briefed to press the issue. In this case, the actor–patient would have been briefed to leave the appointment with a script for her PPI, a follow-up blood test, some information on treatments for the menopause and a strategy for tackling her on-going calf pain/sciatica. An acceptable strategy would be *"let's discuss this further at a follow-up appointment, which you can arrange, at your convenience, with the receptionist."*

Revising data gathering

What questions could the doctor ask to discover the patient's ideas, and expectations? How could the doctor address the patient's concerns and health beliefs?
- Ideas: *"You mention making a list to help you remember? What do you think is making you forgetful? Do you think that feeling low and lacking energy is due to the menopause?"*
- Concerns: *"Your calf pain sounds like on-going sciatica – nerve pain, rather than a DVT. HRT affects the blood and slightly increases the risk of clotting in the veins. HRT should not make your nerve pain worse and your sciatica does not increase your risk of clotting."*
- Expectations: *"Your list allows us to prioritise things so we can tackle them logically. If we can't get through everything, please remind me that I definitely have to discuss your blood results; what do you definitely have to leave with today?"*
- Health beliefs: *"I agree that your symptoms sound like the menopause. How we treat the menopause depends on which symptoms are troubling you most. HRT is probably better for the lack of energy and irregular bleeding, but if we have reservations about using HRT in you, the low mood and hot flushes could be treated with Prozac-type medication while poor sleep could be treated with regular exercise or valerian. Let me briefly outline each option for you and then give you some written information. How does that sound?"*

Relevant literature

patient.info/doctor/hoarseness-pro

https://cks.nice.org.uk/menopause

tinyurl.com/CS3e-Lc19b (*takes you to* cks.nice.org.uk/dyspepsia-proven-gord)

Background information

Davies, M. (2013) Managing challenging interactions with patients. *BMJ Careers.* tinyurl.com/CS3e-Lc19c (*takes you to* http://careers.bmj.com/careers/advice/view-article.html?id=20013822)

Handling a challenging interaction
Identify that you are in the midst of a difficult consultation, by becoming aware of your stress or other negative feelings.

Resist making subconscious changes in behaviour, such as body language and degree of listening. Try not to argue, talk over the patient, or interrupt the patient as this could lead to a downward spiral in the interaction.

Verbalise the difficulty with the patient. For example, you might say: 'We both have different views on how much can be accomplished within the time constraints of today's consultation and that may cause some difficulty between us. However, we both want you to get the medical help you need to feel better. Do you agree?'

Listen carefully and show empathy. People are more likely to feel supported if they feel that they have been listened to.

Find common ground. 'I agree with you that HRT is not the only option. We could use other treatments including herbal medicines, as you suggested.'

Work together with the patient to find a solution and act in their best interests. A solution-focused process demonstrates that you are working in partnership with the patient.

Long case 20 - Dyspepsia

Brief to the doctor

Mr ST, a 45 year old man, has seen you twice in the past 3 months for dyspepsia. One month ago you gave him a prescription for omeprazole 20 mg once daily for 28 days.

Patient summary

Name	ST
Date of birth (Age)	45
Social and family history	Married
Past medical history	3 months ago: GP consultation: "*4months' dyspepsia. No red flags. Smokes 15/day. Alc – 18 units/week. Intermittent diclofenac for back. OTC Gaviscon helps. OE - NAD. Advised – lose weight, stop smoking, no late meals. Stop diclofenac. Gaviscon prn 500mls.*"
	1 month ago: GP consultation: "*Above not helped. Had partic bad episode and OTC ranitidine helped. Back is OK with paracetamol. Still smoking. Has lost some wt – congratulated. Abdo soft. No red flags, so 1m trial PPI. Omeprazole 20mg od ×28. Rev 1m*"
Current medication	Omeprazole 20 mg od
	Diclofenac 50 mg 1 tds prn for back pain

Investigations	3months ago:
BMI	29.3
BP	134/86
Tobacco	15/day
Alcohol	18 units/wk

Tasks for the doctor

In this case, the tasks are to:
1. ascertain Mr ST's response to the PPI trial
2. agree a management plan including lifestyle changes

Brief to the patient – more about the patient

1. Profile:

- Mr ST is 45 years old. He works in the planning department at the local council. He married with 3 teenage children
- His father died 10 years ago of an MI aged 60; mother alive, hypertensive
- Smokes 15/day – he has tried patches and gum in the past, but was never cigarette free for more than 3 weeks
- drinks 18 units/week (wine)

2. He is seeing the doctor today because:

- he has had indigestion for 7 months – the response to omeprazole has been 'miraculous'
- he would like to continue taking the tablets

3. Additional information:

- If the doctor asks specifically:
  - his indigestion symptoms are: upper abdominal pain between meals with some belching. The pain has woken him at night a couple of times in the past. Symptoms worse after big or late meals. No nausea, vomiting, haematemesis, heartburn, dysphagia.
  - he has lost a few pounds
  - he still gets intermittent back pain, but since being told to stop taking diclofenac, he has been able to control this reasonably well with paracetamol and exercises. He thinks this has been a good move, because it has made him do his exercises and watch his posture rather than 'just take a tablet and mask the pain'.
  - he is not concerned he has anything other than plain indigestion and he does not want any investigations
  - he has heard about *H. pylori* and wonders whether he should be tested as this might give him life-long cure
- He enjoys smoking and finds it helps him relax. If the doctor can present him with evidence that he has other risk factors for heart disease, he might be persuaded to give stopping another try.
- He could easily be persuaded to lose weight and change his diet.
- He would like to be more physically active and is open to suggestions on how to lead a more physically active life. He drives to work, dropping the children off at school on the way. They live on the edge of town, just too far to walk into town easily.

Approach to be taken

A. Data gathering, examination and clinical assessment skills

1. Define the clinical problem: clarify why the patient has presented today
The doctor:
- reads the patient information provided prior to the consultation
- asks open questions to explore how Mr ST responded to the omeprazole and whether he believes the lifestyle changes he made previously helped: *"How have things been since I saw you last?"*
- asks closed questions to exclude red flag symptoms signalling the need for referral
- discovers Mr ST's desire to keep taking omeprazole: *"Have you any ideas about what we should do now?"*
- clarifies whether Mr ST would like further tests: *"Have you heard about any investigations or tests for this?"*

2. Performs an appropriate physical or mental examination
- In this case, an examination is not required.

B. Clinical management skills

3. Make an appropriate working diagnosis
- The doctor, based on the history, makes a working diagnosis of uninvestigated dyspepsia with no red flags; Mr ST tells you that he is happy with this diagnosis.

4. Explain the problem to the patient using appropriate language
The doctor:
- having quickly established Mr ST's response to omeprazole, addresses his agenda: wanting to keep taking omeprazole
- provides some information on the effectiveness of lifestyle changes in the management of dyspepsia

5. Provide holistic care and use resources effectively
The doctor:
- informs Mr ST about *H. pylori* testing, eradication treatment and success rates and ascertains whether he would like to explore this treatment option
- discusses the pros and cons of using omeprazole long-term, either continuously or intermittently
- explores Mr ST's ideas about smoking and the benefits of stopping smoking: *"Have you any thoughts about how smoking might be affecting you?"*
- identifies other risk factors for CVD: FH, overweight, relative lack of exercise and uses this to try to motivate Mr ST to stop smoking, lose weight and lead a more physically active lifestyle

- congratulates Mr ST for managing his back pain without diclofenac – this is an opportunity to reinforce a message that self-management can be very effective

6. *Prescribe appropriately*
The doctor:
- is aware of national and local guidelines – NICE guideline CG184 (2014) *Dyspepsia and gastro-oesophageal reflux disease*; see tinyurl.com/CS3e-Lc20a (*takes you to* https://pathways.nice.org.uk/pathways/dyspepsia-and-gastro-oesophageal-reflux-disease/...)
- negotiates an appropriate treatment option:
  - ○ return to self-management (as per NICE guidelines)
  - ○ intermittent PPI use
  - ○ *H. pylori* testing
- offers smoking cessation advice
- offers advice on diet, weight loss and increased physical activity

7. *Specify the conditions and interval for follow-up*
The doctor:
- signposts Mr ST to information on CVD risk factors
- offers a follow-up appointment either with a doctor or with a nurse to discuss smoking cessation and other lifestyle modifications
- arranges a follow up appointment to review the *H. pylori* test result
- safety nets – informs Mr ST about dyspepsia 'red-flag' symptoms
- confirms understanding – *"To summarise, we discussed* H.pylori *testing, lifestyle changes and long-term treatment with omeprazole. What points have you taken away from our discussion?"*

C. Interpersonal skills: know and treat this patient

8. *Achieve rapport*
The doctor:
- listens actively and explores the patient's health ideas, concerns and expectations
- in particular, explores and clarifies Mr ST's beliefs about medication, smoking and motivation for stopping smoking
- explores ways to motivate the patient to lose weight and to become more physically active
- displays empathy and is non-judgemental about Mr ST's weight and smoking

9. *Give the patient the opportunity to be involved in significant management decisions*
The doctor:
- actively confirms the patient's understanding of the dyspepsia and CVD risk factors: *"Does all this make sense to you?"*
- shares thoughts and involves patient in deciding which management option to select

- encourages autonomy and opinions – provides him with information so he feels able to understand self-management for himself and his family
- supports and congratulates his self-management of his back pain

Debrief

Discuss how the doctor could, if needed, improve his performance. In particular, assess how the doctor:

- negotiated an appropriate management plan for dyspepsia
- discussed CVD risk factors
- tried to motivate Mr ST to stop smoking
- structured the consultation and used the time appropriately

Revising data gathering

What questions could the doctor ask to discover the patient's ideas, concerns, expectations and health beliefs?

- Ideas: "*I understand that you are keen to continue on omeprazole; have you thought about other ways to treat your symptoms?*"
- Concerns: "*You don't seem keen on stopping smoking. Are there any particular reasons?*"
- Expectations: "*It seems that you are not very happy with your current diet; would you like to discuss how it could be improved?*"
- Health beliefs: "*You know that smoking increases your risk of heart disease, but there are other factors as well. Would you like to check over these and see if any apply to you?*"

Relevant literature

Delaney BC, Qume M, Moayyedi P, *et al.* (2008) *Helicobacter pylori* test and treat versus proton pump inhibitor in initial management of dyspepsia in primary care: multicentre randomised controlled trial (MRC-CUBE trial). *BMJ,* **336:** 651–654.

NICE (2014) *Dyspepsia and GORD* (CG184): www.nice.org.uk/guidance/cg184

Background information

Ford, A.C. and Moayyedi, P. (2013) Dyspepsia. *BMJ*, **347**: f5059. www.bmj.com/content/347/bmj.f5059

Clinical review: Dyspepsia

Gastro-oesophageal cancer is extremely rare in patients with dyspepsia who have no alarm symptoms, such as

- Age ≥55 years with new onset dyspepsia
- Chronic gastrointestinal bleeding
- Dysphagia
- Progressive unintentional weight loss
- Persistent vomiting
- Iron deficiency anaemia
- Epigastric mass
- Suspicious barium meal result

Dyspepsia describes pain or discomfort (for at least 3 months) in the epigastric region – it is a symptomatic diagnosis. GORD is reserved for patients with predominantly heartburn or regurgitation.

Dyspepsia is more common in people who take non-steroidal anti-inflammatory drugs (NSAIDs), calcium antagonists, bisphosphonates, nitrates and theophyllines, and in those infected with *Helicobacter pylori*. Dyspepsia is also associated with anxiety.

About 5% of dyspepsia in the community is attributable to *H. pylori*. In patients who are *H. pylori* negative, and who are not taking NSAIDs, peptic ulcer disease is rare and probably requires long-term PPI treatment.

Doctors often advise people with dyspepsia to lose weight, avoid fatty food and alcohol, or stop smoking, but there is little evidence that these measures improve symptoms. As a result, drugs are the mainstay of treatment.

There is increasing evidence that tricyclic antidepressants, but not selective serotonin reuptake inhibitors, are beneficial in functional dyspepsia but there is no evidence that psychological treatments (such as CBT), are beneficial.

Preparing for the MRCGP Clinical Skills Assessment (CSA)

In this section, we shall discuss:

- how to use the practice cases, including
  - the 'patient'
  - the 'doctor'
  - the 'examiner'
  - the usefulness of these scenarios for group CSA practice
- information about the CSA, including:
  - the structure of the CSA
  - what happens on the exam day
  - the marking of the CSA
  - preparing for the CSA

How to use the practice cases

The following practice cases will help GP trainees prepare for Clinical Skills Assessment (CSA). They are written for use in a study group, ideally consisting of three trainees.

Please note that some of the practice cases were originally published in *GP*, and are reproduced here with permission (www.gponline.com).

The 'patient'
The trainee playing the 'patient' should read the 'brief to the patient' section to enable her to understand the expectations of the patient so she can then answer the doctor's questions. If an examination is expected, the patient is briefed about the findings and may have to make up a card containing the relevant information prior to starting the consultation. If the patient brief does not contain this information, for example a BP reading, and the doctor wishes to examine the patient, the patient should allow the examination to actually occur. Performing irrelevant or unjustified examinations eats into the consultation time. If the 'doctor' asks to perform intimate examinations not contained within the patient brief, the patient should decline.

The 'doctor'
The 'doctor' should read the 'patient medical record' section at the start of the consultation because it contains a summary of the patient's relevant details. A recent test result, such as a fasting glucose result, may be provided. Sometimes, a copy of the last patient consultation is given. The background information often provides a clue about today's consultation or gives important data relevant to today's management decisions.

The 'examiner'

Ideally, the third trainee playing the 'examiner' should enter the consulting room with the patient and sit unobtrusively where the 'doctor' cannot see him. The examiner should mark the case using the 'marking guide' by ticking against the positive or negative indicators as the consultation unfolds. At the end of the consultation, the examiner should also make a global judgement of whether the 'doctor', based on this consultation, is fit for independent practice. The 'examiner' times the case, sounding an alarm when the ten minutes are up.

The usefulness of these scenarios for group CSA practice

The CSA tests the candidate's ability to gather and assess medical information, make structured, evidence-based and flexible decisions and communicate with patients in a way that moves the consultation forward in an ethical and responsible manner. The candidate passes if he or she is able to ask the patient the right questions, at the right time, in the right way, perform the right examination correctly and communicate effectively, all within ten minutes. The marking grid in each practice case for CSA study groups provides the model for an ordered, step-wise approach to data gathering, management and communication. However, the group debrief, using the debrief prompts at the end of each case, is essential to review the actual performance. The group feedback informs the doctor about his current knowledge and communication skills and advises him on how he can improve his performance for success in the CSA.

Information about the CSA

The structure of the CSA

The CSA is one of the three components of the MRCGP assessment. It is designed to test a doctor's ability to **integrate** and **apply** clinical, professional, communication and practical skills appropriate for general practice, "to produce a consultation that is meaningful to both patient and doctor and which moves the patient forward towards a justifiable management of their presenting problem" (Hawthorne, 2007).

What happens on exam day

- On the day of the examination, at the examination venue, each candidate is given a consulting room.
- The candidate is briefed to treat the examination session as if he is a locum doctor.
- He is to interact with the patient and not the examiner, who will remain a silent observer.
- The candidate's surgery has thirteen booked patients who enter his consulting room when the buzzer sounds.
- At the end of 10 minutes, the buzzer sounds to signal the departure of the patient.
- There is a two minute gap between consultations.
- Twelve patients are true examination cases on which the candidate is assessed. One is a 'trial station' in which new clinical scenarios are trialled. The candidate will not know which is the trial case.
- There will be a short break in the middle of surgery.

The marking of CSA

The patients, played by trained actors, will move from room to room, together with the examiner for that case. Each examiner will mark the same case all day, thus providing standardised marking.

Each case is marked in three domains, and all have equal weighting.

- *Data gathering, examination and clinical assessment skills*: the ability to take a targeted history and perform a focused physical examination. Candidates are expected to be knowledgeable and skilful in their examination techniques and in the appropriate use of medical instruments. Marks are awarded for the fluency with which procedures are performed.
- *Clinical management skills*: in line with current accepted British general practice.
- *Interpersonal skills:* the candidate shows an ability to engage patients in the consultation, using recognised interpersonal skills, such as enquiring about the patient's health beliefs and incorporating these into the explanation given to the patient. Some cases also assess the candidate's ability to value patients' contributions, and to respect their autonomy and decision-making.

The pass mark is set as the standard required to practise independently as a licensed GP. The candidate is then given an overall grade, namely a Clear Pass, Marginal Pass, Marginal Fail or Clear Fail.

In very simple terms, data-gathering is about *how* you get to the 'nub' of the presenting problem; clinical management is about *what* you do to move the problem forward; and interpersonal skills is about *how* you go about doing it.

Each case is written to focus on a particular 'nub'. The marking schedule, using positive and negative indicators of practice, reflects this nub. Please refer to video cases 8 to 13 for examples of the marking schedule.

Preparing for CSA

Do the job. The CSA cases are all written by GPs active in the UK National Health Service and reflect real-life presentations. Therefore, candidates with some experience in NHS general practice should not have difficulty with the exam. The RCGP recommends that candidates first complete at least 6 months of UK NHS GP practice before sitting the exam.

Read the website. Candidates are advised to read the Curriculum Statements from the RCGP website. Each curriculum statement has a section on common and important conditions and cases are quite likely to be based on one of these.

Analyse your consultations. Candidates are advised to video their own consultations, watch them with a colleague, and analyse them for the clinical approach and interpersonal skills displayed. Alternatively, candidates may work in small groups, practising cases such as the ones contained in this section of the book.

Practise clinical examinations. Candidates are advised to practise the focused examinations that are most likely to be tested, such as assessment of a limb, chest or abdomen. Some examinations, such as intimate examinations on a role player, or examinations that might cause discomfort if repeated, are less likely to be tested. Candidates are advised to be familiar and confident with medical equipment, such as otoscopes.

Interpret data. Candidates are advised to become familiar with the letters GPs receive from secondary care, and test results such as ECGs, spirometry, blood tests, urinalysis, skin scrapings and swabs. Candidates need to ensure that they can interpret results correctly and explain them to a patient.

The practice CSA cases in this section of the book include cases that require candidates to practise physical examination and interpret test results.

Additional reading

Malik S (2006) An OSCE actress. *BMJ Career Focus,* **332**: 110.

Ms Malik describes her experience as an OCSE actress, how she was briefed to play the case, and what examiners asked of her regarding the candidates. She also gives her tips on how candidates should prepare:

> "I would suggest that if you can sense the acting patient is not happy with the situation then you should ask: "*Is there anything I've said that is confusing or not clear or that you want explained again?*" Another tip is to have a mental checklist of questions prepared and if you find yourself in an awkward situation, go back to where you left off in the list."

Relevant literature

Hawthorne K (2007) Introduction to the cases in the Clinical Skills Assessment. RCGP website: www.rcgp-curriculum.org.uk/nmrgcp/csa/csa_cases.aspx

Simpson RG (2007) Preparing for practice: nMRCGP and the Clinical Skills Assessment. *Update,* **75**: 36–37.

Royal College of General Practitioners MRCGP website: www.rcgp.org.uk/-/media/Files/GP-training-and-exams/Annual-reports/MRCGP-Fairness-Report-v010215.ashx?la=en, particularly:
- www.rcgp-curriculum.org.uk/PDF/curr_1_Curriculum_Statement_Being_a_GP.pdf
  for the GP curriculum – the core statement
- www.rcgp.org.uk/GP-training-and-exams/~/media/Files/GP-training-and-exams/Curriculum-2012/RCGP-Curriculum-Introduction-and-User-Guide-2012.ashx
  for in-depth reading of learning outcomes for general practice

Practice case 1 – Child

Brief to the patient

- You are Katie Perret, a 29 year old mum. You present today without your children to obtain a prescription for 2½ year old Anne and to ask for advice about 5 year old Olivia's night terrors.
- When you consulted with Anne ten days ago, the doctor agreed with you that Anne's persistent night-time cough and her occasional wheeze may be caused by asthma. She advised you to try a blue salbutamol inhaler. Anne used the inhaler and the face mask without difficulty. It has made some difference but she is not completely better.
- Anne has used the inhaler 2–3 times per day. Thirty minutes after using the inhaler, her cough recurs. You are not sure if the blue inhaler alone is adequate medication. You have been asthmatic since childhood and based on your experience, you feel Anne needs a brown steroid inhaler.
- You are concerned about the night-time cough. It still disturbs Olivia who has to wake up for school the next morning. You are also worried about Olivia's night terrors. Is the poor sleep making the night terrors worse? Is there anything you could do to help Olivia with her night terrors?
- Olivia has had night terrors from the age of 3. The health visitor advised a good night routine for Olivia, but despite this she tends to get one at least once a week. If questioned, it usually happens two hours after she falls asleep. She sits bolt upright in bed, screams like mad, looks ashen, cries inconsolably and never remembers it in the morning. It is difficult to rouse her in the middle of a terror.
- You would like to get a prescription for a brown steroid inhaler for Anne and some advice for Olivia. You didn't think Anne needed to be re-examined today. She is usually fine during the day and at the last consultation, the doctor did not detect anything untoward on examination. You really don't think it is worth coming back with the children for medication to be issued. If you are asked to return before a prescription is issued, you want to know what the examination will add to the consultation.

Patient medical record for the doctor

Name   Anne Perret (2½ years old)

Consultation note by GP (ten days ago)
'Mum had asthma from age 5. Anne occasionally has cough at night (after 9pm) and over last few nights, mum noticed wheeze. Kept sister (school age) awake. Tried steam inhalation / propping up head of bed, but did not help. Frustrated as presented many

---

times with cough and told it is a self-limiting viral illness. O/E: chest sounds normal; no wheeze. Tearing up surgery, healthy looking. Plan: try salbutamol inhaler and review if needed.'

Marking guide for the assessor

Generic indicators for targeted assessment domains	Descriptors – positive and negative
A. Data gathering, technical and assessment skills: • Gathering of data for clinical judgement, choice of examination, investigations and their interpretations. • Demonstrating proficiency in performing physical examinations and using diagnostic and therapeutic instruments.	Positive indicators: • Reads the previous consultation prior to the patient's presentation. • Asks open questions to clarify the nature of the problem followed by closed questions to understand exactly what mum is requesting today. • The doctor systematically excludes red flags (intercurrent illness; severe asthma) that may signal the need for in-person review. • Comes to an understanding of how Anne's night-time cough exacerbates Olivia's night terrors and the impact on the family. • Elicits mum's concerns about Anne's 'partially treated asthma' and her expectations of a prescription. Negative indicators: • The doctor fails to respond to mum's cues about 'disturbed sleep'. By not establishing the link between disturbed sleep and Olivia's worsening night terrors, the doctor does not provide holistic family care.

B. Clinical management skills • Recognition and management of common medical conditions in primary care. Demonstrates flexible and structured approach to decision-making. • Demonstrating ability to deal with multiple complaints and co-morbidity and to promote a shared approach to managing problems.	Positive indicators: • Makes a clinically sound working diagnosis on the basis of probability. Offers very low to low dose inhaled corticosteroid inhaler (e.g. Clenil Modulite 50µg 2–4 puffs twice daily by pressurised metered dose inhalers with spacer. tinyurl.com/CS3e-Pc1a (*takes you to* www.guidelines.co.uk/btssign/asthma-in-children) • The explanation about interrupted sleep aggravating night terrors is logical and incorporates the patient's beliefs. • Advises about the treatment of night terrors; see UCLH patient information leaflet. • Outlines when follow-up or review is needed (safety-nets). If referral to the asthma nurse is offered (for checking inhaler technique, triggers, compliance), mum is given sufficient information to make a decision. Negative indicators: • Fails to prescribe safely, or in line with current best practice, or fails to justify why a prescription is given or withheld. • Fails to check the patient's understanding of the medication and/or her ability to use the medication appropriately. • Fails to formulate a management plan for night terrors or fails to advise why this needs to be addressed in a separate consultation.

C. Interpersonal skills	Positive indicators:
• Use of recognised communication techniques that enhance understanding of a patient's illness and promote a shared approach to managing problems. • Practising ethically with respect for equality and diversity in line with accepted codes of professional conduct.	• Listens attentively and empathises with adverse effect of nocturnal cough on the family. • Is non-judgemental about mum's ideas; refrains from retorting, 'So you think a steroid inhaler is needed. At which medical school did you train?' • Encourages mum's opinions and autonomy but maintains primary duty of care to the children. Negative indicators: • The doctor interrupts unnecessarily and breaks the flow of conversation. • The doctor's manner discourages questioning or the sharing of opinions. • The patient is not offered options regarding treatment or follow-up.

Group debrief

Discuss how the doctor could, if needed, improve his or her performance.

In particular, assess whether the doctor 'showed poor time management':
• How long did the doctor take to obtain the history? Was questioning efficient, appropriately selective or needlessly repetitive?
• Was the second half of the consultation (clinical management, explaining and follow-up arrangements) rushed?
• Were the relevant psychosocial factors covered?

In the group, discuss whether the doctor developed an adequate management plan:
• What was the management plan? Was it appropriate to the level of risk?
• Were the possible risks and benefits of different management approaches, including prescribing, clearly identified and discussed?

Relevant literature

van Dorp F. (2008) Consultations with children. *InnovAiT*, **1 (1):** 54–61.

Driver H.S. & Shapiro C.M. (1993) ABC of sleep disorders. Parasomnias. *BMJ*, **306:** 921 doi:10.1136/bmj.306.6882.921

tinyurl.com/CS3e-Pc1a (*takes you to* www.guidelines.co.uk/btssign/asthma-in-children)

tinyurl.com/CS3e-Pc1b (*takes you to* www.uclh.nhs.uk/PandV/PIL/...)

Practice case 2 – Adult man

Brief to the patient

- You are Martin Rice, a 41 year old unmarried municipal gardener. You are brought in today by your work colleague Jim, who on visiting your flat, found you wrapped in a duvet and throwing up. You smell of alcohol.
- You present as an emergency. Jim was concerned that you hadn't reported to work after a week of sick leave, which you were given by the consultant psychiatrist last week. The psychiatrist thought your feelings of panic were due to your medication (venlafaxine) being dropped from 75 mg to 37.5 mg, so he increased it back to 75mg once daily and also prescribed some diazepam. You took all the diazepam in the first two days, but because you continued to feel panicky, you drank alcohol.
- Jim confirms that you drank 6 litres of vodka over the week. He found the empty bottles in your room. Unless asked, Jim sits quietly in the room and lets you speak.
- You are adamant that you usually drink hardly any alcohol. You binged over the last six days to self-medicate the anxiety. The medication changes did not touch the anxiety and you 'want help'.
- If asked, you admit to feeling very agitated and your legs feel restless. You have not been sweating excessively. You say you do not have a tremor; you have not had any hallucinations or periods of confusion. You have not been using recreational drugs.
- If questioned about your past history, you have been on venlafaxine for two years to treat depression. About 12 months ago you were admitted to hospital for a brief period when you experienced a similar reaction when your medication was reduced. You barely remember the details, only that the nurses were very rude and you eventually self-discharged because they were not helping you.
- You want further time off work to allow the venlafaxine to work. You want tablets stronger than the diazepam to help your anxiety. If advised that it is not safe for you to go home alone, you say you can go to your mother's house in Stafford. You offer the GP your mother's mobile number. You prefer not to be hospitalised.
- You appear very agitated with fidgety legs and hands throughout the consultation.

Patient medical record for the doctor

Name	Martin Rice (41 years)
Past medical history	Depression (moderate to severe) 2009 Left scaphoid fracture 2005
Current medication	Venlafaxine 37.5 mg once daily

Consultation by patient's usual GP (ten days ago)

'Two weeks ago reduced venlafaxine to 37.5 mg and starting to feel he is in a downward spiral, mood dropped, difficulty focusing at work. Started drinking 2 days ago and turned up to work drunk yesterday. No withdrawals or cravings. No thoughts of DSH. Lives alone. Gets nightmares and struggles to stay asleep. Plan: patient keen to get back to work. Will increase meds back to 75 mg. Advised to throw alcohol away. I will write to psychiatrist to request review appointment brought forward to this week.'

Marking guide for the assessor

Generic indicators for targeted assessment domains	Descriptors – positive and negative
A. Data gathering, technical and assessment skills: • Gathering of data for clinical judgement, choice of examination, investigations and their interpretations. • Demonstrating proficiency in performing physical examinations and using diagnostic and therapeutic instruments.	Positive indicators: • Asks selective questions, tailored to establishing what has triggered the patient's anxiety and restlessness. • Enquires about the medication, possible side effects, dosing regime and compliance. Takes a comprehensive alcohol and drug history. • Enquires about red flags, such as delirium tremens, deliberate self-harm and risk to others from the patient's driving and occupation. Negative indicators: • Questioning and examination is not sufficiently selective. Most questions should address the alcohol issue in order to safely manage the patient's withdrawal symptoms. • The patient's use of diazepam or other drugs and the co-existence of physical or psychiatric illness are not explored. • Details of the patient's support network are not obtained.

B. Clinical management skills	Positive indicators:
• Recognition and management of common medical conditions in primary care. Demonstrates flexible and structured approach to decision-making. • Demonstrating ability to deal with multiple complaints and co-morbidity and to promote a shared approach to managing problems.	• Doctor discusses what they feel is the safest course of action and explain their reasoning. • Management options, including possible hospital admission or management in the community, are openly discussed. • Management is appropriate to the patient's level of risk, the doctor's experience, and the ability to enlist the help of support networks and agencies. • Doctor advises appropriately on work and driving. Negative indicators: • Doctor fails to manage safely or in line with current best practice. • Follow-up arrangements are inadequate.
C. Interpersonal skills	Positive indicators:
• Use of recognised communication techniques that enhance understanding of a patient's illness and promote a shared approach to managing problems. • Practising ethically with respect for equality and diversity in line with accepted codes of professional conduct.	• Doctor displays a good mix of empathy and direction. • He or she communicates effectively with the patient, not his colleague. • Doctor obtains the patient's permission to discuss issues in front of the colleague or with his mother by telephone. • They develop a shared management plan, stressing what is safe management for the patient and others around him (work colleagues / road users) who could be harmed. Negative indicators: • The doctor assumes the patient cannot provide a history and communicates with the work colleague. • The doctor's non-verbal communication and language is doctor-centred, potentially creating a parent–child dynamic. • The doctor appears judgemental about the use of alcohol.

Group debrief

- What questioning or examining enabled the doctor to differentiate between acute alcohol withdrawal, delirium tremens or serotonin discontinuation syndrome? Was the line of questioning methodical or erratic? Was the history taking tailored or did the doctor ask a battery of non-selective, rote psychiatric questions?
- Did the doctor recognise significant findings: such as lack of support at home, co-existing depression and previous self-discharge possibly from in-patient detoxification. How did the doctor use this information to negotiate a safe management plan?
- The most common reason for failure in the CSA is the doctor not developing a management plan (including prescribing and referral) reflecting knowledge of current best practice. Did the doctor manage this patient in line with current UK best practice?
- Doctors with good interpersonal skills actively listen, appear to really want to know the patient's answers, and skilfully weave the patient's ideas, concerns and expectations into their management plan. Assess whether this consultation was doctor- or patient-centred and suggest how it could safely be made more patient-centred.

Relevant literature

NICE (2011) Alcohol use disorders: diagnosis, assessment and management of harmful drinking and alcohol dependence: www.nice.org.uk/guidance/cg115

tinyurl.com/CS3e-Pc2a (*takes you to* www.nice.org.uk/guidance/cg115/resources/...)

Practice case 3 - Baby

Brief to the patient

- You are Paula Hayden, a 25 year old mum. You called the practice to check if your baby's eye swab result has arrived.
- The receptionist informed you that the results are available but she cannot pass them to you. She placed your name in the duty doctor's clinic for him or her to call you back.
- Your baby, Tom, developed sticky eyes when he was five days old. Your GP took a swab and prescribed chloramphenicol eye ointment which you have been using for four days.
- Tom still has sticky eyes but does not seem to be unwell. This morning you noticed a slight streak of blood on his eyelid. You are not sure if this is from scratching, perhaps because of ongoing discomfort. You wanted to check if the 'right' antibiotic was prescribed, hence you called for the swab result.
- You are concerned about Chlamydia eye infection. Your husband had a one-night stand a few months ago. He went to the GUM clinic for treatment and you took antibiotics on their advice. You have read on the internet that Chlamydia can cause conjunctivitis.
- You and your husband have discussed his infidelity. You have forgiven him and believe that he has been faithful since. However, you are concerned about Tom and angry that he is 'suffering' from an eye infection.
- If questioned, Tom was born by vaginal delivery five days after your due date. There were no problems during your pregnancy and labour. His baby check prior to discharge was fine. He feeds well and except for his eye infection, you have no concerns.
- You are happy to bring Tom for a doctor's appointment later today. You plan to travel to your mum's house in North Wales early tomorrow morning. You will be on holiday for two weeks. You would prefer to get any 'new' antibiotics from your GP before you leave. You are not keen to take your baby to the GUM clinic.

Patient medical record for the doctor

Name   Tom Hayden (9 days old)

Note by receptionist (today)
Mum (Paula) called for eye swab result. Advised that duty doctor will call her later on 07744 226688. Telephone appointment made.

This practice case originally appeared in *GP* and is reproduced here in an amended form with permission (see **www.gponline.com**)

Specimen   Eye swab (today)

Chlamydia PCR *C. trachomatis* DNA detected (CDR). Patient and partner STD screening available at GUM. Patients may telephone directly for an appointment on 0745 910 3355.

Consultation note by GP (four days ago)
'Developed bilateral sticky eyes 5 days ago. Parents concerned about Chlamydia – openly discussed. Swab taken. Chloramphenicol prescribed.'

Marking guide for the assessor

Generic indicators for targeted assessment domains	Descriptors – positive and negative
A. Data gathering, technical and assessment skills: • Gathering of data for clinical judgement, choice of examination, investigations and their interpretations. • Demonstrating proficiency in performing physical examinations and using diagnostic and therapeutic instruments.	Positive indicators: • Establishes the identity of the caller and patient. • Asks open questions to clarify the nature of the problem followed by closed questions to understand exactly what the mum is requesting today. • The doctor systematically excludes red flags signalling the need for in-person review or referral. This is important; the difficulty with telephone triage is the ability to make management decisions in the absence of visual cues. With ophthalmia neonatorum (ON), you expect to get a history of conjunctival redness, discharge and swelling of the lids (distinguish between simple sticky eyes and conjunctival inflammation). In addition, the cornea may be involved (especially with *N. gonorrhoeae*) with possible corneal perforation, which is the reason for needing urgent ophthalmology assessment. The child with chlamydia ON is also at risk of developing pneumonia.

	Negative indicators:
	• It would be difficult to do a telephone consultation, especially one on a sensitive topic, without first establishing identity and rapport. • The doctor fails to read and understand the medical information provided prior to phoning. • The doctor fails to elicit the patient's concerns about Chlamydia before discussing the swab results. • The doctor fails to elicit the patient's expectation for new antibiotics.
B. Clinical management skills • Recognition and management of common medical conditions in primary care. Demonstrates flexible and structured approach to decision-making. • Demonstrating ability to deal with multiple complaints and co-morbidity and to promote a shared approach to managing problems.	Positive indicators: • Treats Chlamydia eye infection in line with current guidance: referral to ophthalmology and erythromycin 50 mg/kg/day in 4 divided doses. Topical treatment is not required. • Gives information about Chlamydia eye infection and sexual health in digestable chunks. The patient's understanding is checked at each step. • Management addresses Mrs Hayden's concerns and expectations. • Outlines when follow-up or review is needed (safety-nets). • Summarises well and ends with 'Are you happy with these arrangements?' Negative indicators: • Doctors fail to refer and/or prescribe safely or in line with current best practice. • Chlamydia and marital issues are not explored holistically. • Follow-up arrangements are inadequately discussed.

C. Interpersonal skills	Positive indicators:
• Use of recognised communication techniques that enhance understanding of a patient's illness and promote a shared approach to managing problems. • Practising ethically with respect for equality and diversity in line with accepted codes of professional conduct.	• Listens attentively to Mrs Hayden's request for advice regarding Tom's ongoing eye symptoms. • Questions in a systematic manner but takes care not to 'interrogate' the patient. • Explores her request for advice from the duty doctor today and refrains from making comments such as 'Why couldn't you wait for your GP to call you?' Negative indicators: • The doctor interrupts unnecessarily and breaks the flow of conversation. • The doctor lacks sensitivity in his or her queries regarding Chlamydia and marital issues. • The doctor fails to encourage autonomy and opinions. The patient is not offered options regarding treatment or follow-up.

Group debrief

Discuss how the doctor could, if needed, improve his or her performance. In particular, assess whether the doctor:

- gathered sufficient data to distinguish between simple sticky eyes and conjunctival inflammation requiring referral to secondary care?
- established rapport on the telephone? If so, how?
- established Mrs Hayden's reasons for calling, her specific concerns and expectations? If so, how?
- summarised and checked understanding?

A common reason for failure in the CSA is that the doctor 'does not identify the patient's agenda, health beliefs and preferences or does not make use of verbal and non-verbal cues'. In the group, discuss what specific questions the doctor could ask to discover the patient's ideas, concerns, expectations and health beliefs? Do these questions blend into the conversation? Which questions sound out-of-place, as if asked by rote? If the questions sound clunky, how would you rephrase them?

Relevant literature

For guidance on management see: tinyurl.com/CS3e-Pc3a (*takes you to* https://cks.nice.org.uk/conjunctivitis-infective#!scenario:2)

For guidance on telephone consultations, see
Car J. & Sheikh A. (2003) Telephone consultations. *BMJ*, **326:** 966–969; doi:10.1136/bmj.326.7396.966. Box 2 on page 968 is useful.

Practice case 4 – Adult woman

Brief to the patient

- You are Mariam Aziz, a 71 year old pensioner. Today you travelled from Glasgow to visit your son and his family.
- You present as an emergency because you forgot to pack your blood pressure medication.
- Your son called your Glasgow practice and spoke to the receptionist who read out the list of medication on your repeat script, namely bendroflumethiazide 2.5 mg once daily, atenolol 50 mg once daily, aspirin 75 mg once daily, and diazepam 2 mg at night.
- Your son accompanies you into the consultation to introduce you to his GP and because he has the list of medication.
- You speak good English. If asked, you don't mind your son coming in with you. However, if probed about your medical issues, you become uncomfortable discussing these in your son's presence and would prefer that the doctor ask him to leave the room.
- When you give the doctor the list of medication, you mention that a week ago, the hospital heart doctor recently added a tablet because the heart was 'getting weaker'. You are unable to remember the tablet's name. Your feet are not swollen and your pulse today is 64 bpm and regular.
- If questioned about the diazepam in front of your son, you are reluctant to discuss the issue. If on your own, you discuss your grief at your husband's death two years ago, your subsequent depression and insomnia. You stopped the anti-depressants but when you tried stopping the diazepam, you felt anxious and couldn't sleep. The psychiatrist advised that you continue with a small dose of diazepam at night. You want the diazepam prescribed and become upset and challenge the doctor if he or she seems reluctant to prescribe it.
- You are happy for the doctor to call your GP and issue a script later.
- You come across as a quiet, unassuming woman but when asked, you have opinions on what you want.
- You are also slightly hard of hearing and if the doctor speaks too quietly (or too rapidly), you ask him or her to repeat the information.

Patient medical record for the doctor

Name   Mariam Aziz (71 years)

Past medical history   Not known – patient is a temporary resident

---

This practice case originally appeared in *GP* and is reproduced here in an amended form with permission (see **www.gponline.com**)

Marking guide for the assessor

Generic indicators for targeted assessment domains	Descriptors – positive and negative
A. Data gathering, technical and assessment skills: • Gathering of data for clinical judgement, choice of examination, investigations and their interpretations. • Demonstrating proficiency in performing physical examinations and using diagnostic and therapeutic instruments.	Positive indicators: • Establishes rapport with Mrs Aziz and is mindful of discussing her medical issues in front of her son. • Asks open questions (to explore the medication request) followed by closed questions to clarify how the list was compiled and whether the repeat script includes the 'new' tablet. • Enquires about the medication, possible side effects, dosing regime and compliance. • Excludes red flags, such as heart failure or arrhythmias. Negative indicators: • Questioning is not sufficiently detailed. Most questions should address a medication review to enable safe prescribing. • The patient's use of diazepam is not explored. • If a physical examination is undertaken, examination skills are neither sufficiently selective nor fluent.

B. Clinical management skills	Positive indicators:
• Recognition and management of common medical conditions in primary care. Demonstrates flexible and structured approach to decision-making. • Demonstrating ability to deal with multiple complaints and co-morbidity and to promote a shared approach to managing problems.	• Doctors discuss what they feel is the safest course of action and explain their reasoning. • Management options, including writing a script following a telephone call to the patient's GP, are openly discussed and offered to the patient. • Management is appropriate to the patient's level of risk. If new medication is to be prescribed, the need for follow-up is discussed. Negative indicators: • Doctors fail to prescribe safely or in line with current best practice. The ongoing need for aspirin 75 mg OD is not explored. • Follow-up arrangements are inadequately discussed.
C. Interpersonal skills	Positive indicators:
• Use of recognised communication techniques that enhance understanding of a patient's illness and promote a shared approach to managing problems. • Practising ethically with respect for equality and diversity in line with accepted codes of professional conduct.	• Doctors display rapport-building skills; they communicate effectively with the patient, not her son, using appropriate language and volume. • Doctors identify the patient's embarrassment at discussing her medical details in front of her son and respond appropriately. • They develop a *shared* management plan, which incorporates the patient's specific concerns about diazepam withdrawal. Negative indicators: • The doctor assumes the patient cannot speak English and communicates with her son. • The language is not pitched at the right level for this patient. • The doctor repeatedly speaks too softly or too loudly. • The doctor appears judgemental about the use of diazepam.

Group debrief

- Assess the doctor's verbal and non-verbal response to the patient and her son. Were assumptions made about the patient based on her ethnic or cultural background?
- Was the patient's medical confidence preserved?
- Was the doctor respectful?
- Did the doctor seem genuinely interested in helping the patient obtain her medication and in prescribing safely?
- Was the patient given the opportunity and time to answer questions?
- Was there a shared management plan that incorporated the patient's concerns and expectations?
- A common reason for failure in the CSA is that the doctor 'does not identify the patient's agenda, health beliefs and preferences or does not make use of verbal and non-verbal cues'. Did the doctor detect and respond to the patient becoming uncomfortable with detailed questioning in her son's presence?
- Another common reason for failure is that the doctor 'does not recognise the challenge' (e.g. the patient's problem or ethical dilemma). Evaluate whether the doctor was mindful of the recent cardiology recommendation and checked if this had been added to the patient's repeat medication. Evaluate whether the patient's medical confidence was protected throughout the consultation.

Relevant literature

For guidance on undertaking medication reviews, see tinyurl.com/CS3e-Pc4a (*takes you to* www.bmj.com/content/bmj/329/7463/434.full.pdf?maxtoshow=&HITS=10&hits=10&RESULTF=)

Practice case 5 – Adult man

Brief to the patient

- You are Rodney Heron, a 33 year old married telecommunications engineer. You present today because you had one of the worst night's sleep earlier this week and want advice on insomnia.
- On Sunday you went to bed at 11 pm, your usual time. You finally dozed off at 3 am. After 3–4 hours of sleep, you felt incredibly tired at work. This is becoming an increasingly common occurrence. You worry about not being able to fall asleep, waking up unrefreshed and feeling tired at work. You haven't made any errors at work but you double-check things now so jobs take longer.
- If asked, the problem started insidiously, about two years ago. Nothing happened to trigger the problem; it just developed. You have poor sleep about three or four nights out of seven. You have difficulty getting off to sleep, but once asleep you are fine. You wake up once to use the toilet, but fall asleep within minutes of returning to bed. You do not have any physical discomforts that wake you.
- You reduced your caffeine intake, you exercise early each evening and you keep the bedroom cool and dark.
- You think your mattress may be too hard (you slept better on holiday 2 weeks ago) but purchasing a new mattress would strain your budget at present. You are not keen on medication; colleagues have warned you how addictive sleeping tablets can be. You want some information so that you can decide if it is safe to try Nytol.
- If asked, you are not depressed; your mood is normal. Your wife has not told you that you have odd or loud breathing sounds or agitated movements when you sleep.
- Two years ago, after your dad had a heart attack, you lost 2 stone, gave up smoking and restricted your alcohol intake to 2 bottles of wine over weekends. It is important to you to maintain a healthy lifestyle. You are not obese and your collar size is 15.
- You want to understand why your sleeping has been affected. If the doctor suggests medication, you want to know the risk of addiction. If asked, you are open to alternative treatments; perhaps these are safer than prescription tablets.

Patient medical record for the doctor

Name	Rodney Heron (33 years)
Past medical history	Surgery for bilateral bunions 2008 Obesity due to excess calories 2006
Current medication	None

This practice case originally appeared in *GP* and is reproduced here in an amended form with permission (see www.gponline.com)

Marking guide for the assessor

Generic indicators for targeted assessment domains	Descriptors – positive and negative
A. Data gathering, technical and assessment skills: • Gathering of data for clinical judgement, choice of examination, investigations and their interpretations. • Demonstrating proficiency in performing physical examinations and using diagnostic and therapeutic instruments.	Positive indicators: • Asks open questions about the sleeping problem, daytime sleepiness/napping and factors interfering with sleep. • Asks closed questions to clarify details and exclude secondary causes of insomnia: depression, alcohol, drugs, sleep apnoea and parasomnias. • Elicits how the problem affects the patient, his family and his work. • Discovers his health beliefs and expectations. Negative indicators: • Questioning and examination is not sufficiently selective. Does not obtain sufficient information to support a diagnosis of primary insomnia. • Failure to work through a diagnostic sieve and actively exclude secondary causes of insomnia. • Details of the patient's agenda and health beliefs are not obtained or believed. The doctor persists in asking about hidden agendas such as depression despite the patient not reporting symptoms of a mood disorder.

B. Clinical management skills	Positive indicators:
• Recognition and management of common medical conditions in primary care. Demonstrates flexible and structured approach to decision-making. • Demonstrating ability to deal with multiple complaints and co-morbidity and to promote a shared approach to managing problems.	• Doctors discuss what they feel the problem is (primary insomnia) and explain their reasoning, using the patient's ideas and beliefs. • Management options, including 'sleep hygiene', restriction of time in bed, drugs, alternative remedies, are openly discussed. • Management addresses the patient's concerns and expectations. • Doctors advise appropriately on work, including the possible impact of a two-week sleep restriction programme on driving. Negative indicators: • Doctors fail to explain the diagnosis or treatment options in jargon-free language. • The evidence base for various treatments is not provided in a simple format. • The patient is not given sufficient information to make informed decisions. • Follow-up arrangements are inadequate.
C. Interpersonal skills	Positive indicators:
• Use of recognised communication techniques that enhance understanding of a patient's illness and promote a shared approach to managing problems. • Practising ethically with respect for equality and diversity in line with accepted codes of professional conduct.	• Doctors listen attentively and summarise appropriately. • They communicate effectively using the patient's ideas and beliefs. • Doctors involve the patient in decisions, offering choices and encouraging autonomy. Negative indicators: • The doctor assumes the patient wants medication; the patient's understanding of the available options is not explored. • The doctor's repeated questions on depression or drugs create the impression that he or she strongly suspects a hidden agenda. • The doctor is unable to discuss the evidence base in a simple and meaningful way.

Group debrief

- Did the doctor ask sufficient questions in sufficient detail to make a diagnosis of primary insomnia? Did the history-taking feel like an interrogation or a conversation? Did the doctor use rote questions that interrupted the flow of the conversation?
- Did the doctor provide management options? Did he or she discuss the pros and cons of 'sleep hygiene', restriction of time in bed, over the counter medications (sedating antihistamines, melatonin, valerian), hypnotic drugs or sedating antidepressants or antipsychotics?
- Some cases in the CSA appear simple. Have the confidence to explore hidden agendas and if they are not present (in this case, by establishing the patient is not depressed or requesting specific medication for illicit purposes), move on. Have the courage to take the patient at face value, as you would in your consulting room.
- This case tests whether the doctor can discuss management options meaningfully with the patient. Is the doctor comfortable with discussing the evidence base? Is the doctor prepared to talk about complementary medicine? This case was not written to check for 'hidden agendas' so beware of second-guessing the examiner. Treat what is in front of you.

Relevant literature

Aung, D. and Chandalia, P. (2013) The darkest hour: diagnosing and managing insomnia. *InnovAiT*, **6(12):** 745–753.

Falloon K. *et al.* (2011) The assessment and management of insomnia in primary care. *BMJ*, **342:** d2899.

Practice case 6 – Adult woman

Brief to the patient

- You are Amanda Shaw, a 51 year old hospital nurse, divorced and living alone.
- You have come to see the doctor today as an emergency on the advice of your friend, with whom you are spending a few days. Your friend is extremely worried about your low mood.
- You feel 'stressed at work' mainly because the ward manager is piling on loads of work in preparation for a CQC visit in 2 weeks. The manager expects you to carry a clinical and administrative workload and undermines you in front of team members. You feel unable to talk to her because she is abrasive and does not listen.
- If asked specifically, you admit to having a low mood for two months, increasing irritability, crying easily, a loss of confidence, difficulty sleeping, 'panic' and moments when you feel very anxious. You are not suicidal. You have not suffered from depression before.
- If questioned in detail, you admit to stopping your HRT 3 months ago after developing vaginal bleeding. Your hysteroscopy was 'horrible' and you don't want to restart HRT. About once a fortnight you are woken up by hot flushes.
- You think you have 'work stress' and difficulty dealing with it because of your menopausal symptoms.
- You want a sick note for 3 weeks, until after the ward visit, so you can stay with your friend and 'get your head around issues'.
- You are worried that your manager and team will think you are a 'shirker' if you request annual leave but you are also concerned that your lack of concentration will result in errors at work which will cause trouble.
- You do not want medication or a referral. You feel the problem lies with your manager.
- You cry intermittently throughout this consultation.

Patient medical record for the doctor

Name Amanda Shaw (51 years)

Past medical history Not known – patient is a temporary resident

This practice case originally appeared in *GP* and is reproduced here in an amended form with permission (see **www.gponline.com**)

Marking guide for the assessor

Generic indicators for targeted assessment domains	Descriptors – positive and negative
A. Data gathering, technical and assessment skills: • Gathering of data for clinical judgement, choice of examination, investigations and their interpretations. • Demonstrating proficiency in performing physical examinations and using diagnostic and therapeutic instruments.	Positive indicators: • Asks open questions (to explore work issues) followed by closed questions to clarify the extent of depressive symptoms. • Enquires about menopausal symptoms and explores their contribution to today's presentation. • Excludes red flags, such as ongoing postmenopausal bleeding and active suicidal ideation. Negative indicators: • Questioning is not selective. Should question about 'bullying at work'; 'menopausal low mood' should be ruled out. • Too much focus on the bio-medical aspects. • Appears disorganised or fails to explain why certain questions are asked.
B. Clinical management skills • Recognition and management of common medical conditions in primary care. Demonstrates flexible and structured approach to decision-making. • Demonstrating ability to deal with multiple complaints and co-morbidity and to promote a shared approach to managing problems.	Positive indicators: • Doctor explains clearly what they feel is the appropriate diagnosis and verbalises their reasoning to the patient. • Management options, including occupational advice, are openly discussed and offered to the patient. • Management, including any prescription, is appropriate to the patient's level of risk. Negative indicators: • Fails to make an adequate diagnosis, namely 'mild to moderate depression with a low suicide risk'. • Management plans, including prescribing, are not appropriate or in line with current best practice. • Follow-up arrangements are inadequate.

C. Interpersonal skills	Positive indicators:
• Use of recognised communication techniques that enhance understanding of a patient's illness and promote a shared approach to managing problems. • Practising ethically with respect for equality and diversity in line with accepted codes of professional conduct.	• Displays good listening skills; identifies the patient's dilemma and fears. • Develops a *shared* management plan, which incorporates the patient's specific concerns about work. • Time off work and follow-up is skilfully negotiated. Negative indicators: • Interrupts inappropriately; appears judgemental or doctor-centred. • Formulaic questions are employed; the questioning on depressive symptoms sounds like a reading of a questionnaire. • Fails to empathise with how this problem has changed the patient's life and her self-perception.

Group debrief

- Assess the doctor's verbal and non-verbal response to the patient's request for a 'sick note'. Did the doctor seem genuinely interested and respectful? Was touch used overly and out of context?
- Was the consultation 'clunky' and lacking in natural flow? Were rote questions and phrases used? Was the patient given time to answer questions? Were questions replicated and old ground covered repeatedly? Did the doctor feel confident, once sufficient data were gathered for a diagnosis, to move smoothly on to management?
- Was there a shared management plan that incorporated the patient's concerns and expectations?
- The most common reason for failure in the CSA is that the doctor 'does not develop a management plan (including prescribing and referral) that is appropriate and in line with current best practice or make adequate arrangements for follow-up and safety-netting'. Evaluate whether the management of this case (mild–moderate depression) was correct, safe and broad enough to eliminate the differential (menopause)?

Relevant literature

McAvoy, B.R. (2003) Workplace bullying. *BMJ*, **326:** 776.
tinyurl.com/CS3e-Pc6a (*takes you to* www.bmj.com/...)

For advice on bullying from the Advisory, Conciliation and Arbitration Service (ACAS), see tinyurl.com/CS3e-Pc6b (*takes you to* www.acas.org.uk/...articleid=1864)

Practice case 7 – Adult woman

Brief to the patient

- You are Evelyn Baker, a 35 year old housewife.
- You present today to discuss the results of a recent blood test. If questioned in detail, you had the 'pre-diabetes test' because a fasting glucose test two months ago showed you had borderline diabetes. You also requested your cholesterol be checked because you are hoping to stop the cholesterol medication.
- You deliberately, without telling the doctor, did not take your cholesterol tablets for one month preceding the blood test in the hope that if the level is low, your doctor will stop the cholesterol tablet. You give this information to the doctor only when your blood results are being discussed.
- With your diet and exercise programme over the last year, you lost a stone and hope a healthy lifestyle will enable you to discontinue medication. You do not experience side effects from medication.
- You think that you may develop diabetes in future. Your mother's parents developed late onset diabetes in their forties. Your father had a heart attack in his fifties and your mother had one in her sixties. Three of your mother's uncles and her only sister have high cholesterol.
- You expect the doctor to discuss your results and to stop the tablets if your cholesterol is low. You also expect your medication for heavy periods to be re-issued today. The gynaecologist you saw two weeks ago advised an operation to burn out the lining of the womb but until then, you need medication to ease the bleeding.
- You are worried about being lectured about further weight loss. You think you have 'big bones' and a 'slow metabolism' and it took enormous effort to lose weight over the last year. You are tired of being warned about the risks of being overweight. You are a non-smoker. You and your husband share three bottles of white wine each week.
- If the doctor offers further blood tests or referral to a specialist, you want to know why.

Patient medical record for the doctor

Name   Evelyn Baker (35 years)

Past medical history   Iron deficiency anaemia 2008
                            Menorrhagia 2008
                            Latex allergy 2007

This practice case originally appeared in *GP* and is reproduced here in an amended form with permission (see **www.gponline.com**)

Current medication	Simvastatin 40 mg at night
	Mefenamic acid 500 mg three times daily
	Tranexamic acid 1 g three times daily

Blood tests	Tests done two weeks ago
HbA1c	6.3% (45 mmol/mol)
Two-hour glucose	10.8 mmol/l
Serum cholesterol	5.9 mmol/l (three years ago 7.9 mmol/l)
HDL	1.1 mmol/l
Hb	13.9 g/dl
BP	136/86
BMI	34.7

Marking guide for the assessor

Generic indicators for targeted assessment domains	Descriptors – positive and negative
A. Data gathering, technical and assessment skills: • Gathering of data for clinical judgement, choice of examination, investigations and their interpretations. • Demonstrating proficiency in performing physical examinations and using diagnostic and therapeutic instruments.	Positive indicators: • Finds out what the patient already knows about the blood tests and why they were done. • Discusses the patient's ideas about cholesterol and explores her beliefs regarding treatment. Discusses her significant family history (the doctor should suspect familial hypercholesterolaemia if dad had premature CVD <55 yrs or mum had CVD <65 yrs). Discusses her cholesterol of 7.9 from 3 years ago. • Discovers the patient's expectation of discontinuing with simvastatin and obtaining a repeat prescription for menorrhagia medication. • The patient is examined for clinical signs of hypercholesterolaemia (look for tendon xanthoma). Negative indicators: • Does not explore her family history. • Time is wasted on examinations that contribute little to subsequent management plans.

B. Clinical management skills	Positive indicators:
• Recognition and management of common medical conditions in primary care. Demonstrates flexible and structured approach to decision-making. • Demonstrating ability to deal with multiple complaints and comorbidity and to promote a shared approach to managing problems.	• Negotiates and highlights the four main issues: her new diagnosis of impaired glucose tolerance, the possibility of familial hypercholesterolaemia, the risks and benefits of statin therapy (NICE advises high intensity statin), and a brief review of menorrhagia management prior to prescribing. • Addresses her concerns about unnecessary statin intake and manages in line with national policy. • The repeat prescription is issued with clear instructions, in line with national prescribing guidance. • Adequate follow-up is arranged and the doctor checks that the patient understands why future tests or referrals are needed. Negative indicators: • Fails to interpret the results appropriately, or the decision regarding statin therapy is not justified. • Prescribes inappropriately. • Follow-up arrangements are inadequate.
C. Interpersonal skills	Positive indicators:
• Use of recognised communication techniques that enhance understanding of a patient's illness and promote a shared approach to managing problems. • Practising ethically with respect for equality and diversity in line with accepted codes of professional conduct.	• Understands why she discontinued medication prior to the blood test. • Provides information about CV risk in language that is easily understood. Explanations are concise. • Provides opportunities for the patient to seek clarification. • Offers options and involves the patient in management decisions. Negative indicators: • Adopts a 'parent–child' style of consulting. • Delivers standard health promotion advice without tailoring it to this patient's needs.

Group debrief

- The focus of some CSA cases is data interpretation. In this case, the patient's blood results are provided for interpretation. You need to interpret the results correctly. Sometimes candidates interpret the results correctly but then fail to act on them appropriately. Examiners therefore conclude that the candidate did not recognise their significance. It is imperative to deal with abnormal findings safely, in line with national or local guidance to reduce risk.
- When candidates fail to interpret data correctly, they invariably do not make the correct working diagnosis. Making a diagnosis means committing yourself on the basis of the information you have available to you. You need a sound knowledge-base.
- State the diagnosis clearly and explain it to the patient using language that is understandable. The lack of a statement about the diagnosis and a vague summary leaves the examiner wondering whether you have made a diagnosis at all. In this case, evaluate how well the doctor explained pre-diabetes and the possibility of familial hypercholesterolaemia to the patient.
- To assess the doctor's interpersonal skills, consider whether the doctor worked in partnership with the patient, involved her in management decisions, and demonstrated evidence of 'shared understanding' by asking the patient to summarise what she understood?

Relevant literature

Choudhary F., Al-Hadithy H. & Simon C. (2009) Hypercholesterolaemia. *InnovAiT*, **2(12):** 721–31.

Familial hypercholesterolaemia: identification and management (2008) NICE guideline CG71.

tinyurl.com/CS3e-Pc7a (*takes you to* https://pathways.nice.org.uk/pathways/familial-hypercholesterolaemia...)

Simon Broome criteria:
tinyurl.com/CS3e-Pc7b

Practice case 8 – Adult woman

Brief to the patient

- You are Lorraine Brooker, a 28 year old accountant, married and in your tenth week of pregnancy.
- You have come to see the doctor today because you have been troubled by headaches, a cold that won't go away, morning sickness, sluggish bowels and thinning hair. You have written a list of your symptoms. Your opening statement is 'I'm so forgetful these days. I brought a list of problems with me.'
- If asked which symptom is most troublesome, you say all the symptoms are troublesome but the headaches are the worst because they have been present for two weeks, since the onset of your cold. The boring pain behind your right eye affects work. The teeth on the right side of your mouth ache. When questioned in detail, you admit to having hot and cold spells at night, an offensive post-nasal drip and your forehead pain worsens when you bend forward.
- You want to know if it is worth buying £12 acupressure bracelets for the nausea.
- Your bowel pattern has altered from once daily to once every two to three days.
- You have always had fine hair but when your cousin was recently diagnosed with a thyroid problem, you checked the internet for advice.
- You think you have a recurrence of migraine (you had this as a teenager). You are concerned about coping with tax season at work with these headaches.
- You want to discuss all your problems. Medication for the headache and a blood test for thyroid disease is a priority. If asked, you are not allergic to any antibiotics.
- If examined, you do not have a temperature and you are tender over the right eye.

Patient medical record for the doctor

Name Lorraine Brooker (28 years)

Past medical history Currently pregnant
Irritable bowel syndrome

Past medication Mebeverine

This practice case originally appeared in *GP* and is reproduced here in an amended form with permission (see **www.gponline.com**)

Marking guide for the assessor

Generic indicators for targeted assessment domains	Descriptors – positive and negative
A. Data gathering, technical and assessment skills: • Gathering of data for clinical judgement, choice of examination, investigations and their interpretations. • Demonstrating proficiency in performing physical examinations and using diagnostic and therapeutic instruments.	Positive indicators: • Asks open questions (to explore the list's contents) followed by closed questions to clarify details, particularly of the headache. • Enquires about the past history of migraine. Understands how pressures at work (and her cousin's recent diagnosis with thyroid disease) affect her presentation today. • The targeted examination is focused, practised and integrated into the consultation. Negative indicators: • Fails to identify the patient's agenda and preferences. • Makes assumptions (about migraine/minor pregnancy symptoms) and fails to recognise the challenge. • Is disorganised in gathering information.
B. Clinical management skills • Recognition and management of common medical conditions in primary care. Demonstrates flexible and structured approach to decision-making. • Demonstrating ability to deal with multiple complaints and co-morbidity and to promote a shared approach to managing problems.	Positive indicators: • Explains clearly what they want to examine and why. • The risks and benefits of management options, including prescribing, are adequately discussed. • Responses to the patient's concerns and expectations are smoothly woven into the consultation. Negative indicators: • Fails to make an adequate diagnosis, with a vague explanation to patient. • Management plans, including prescribing, are not appropriate or in line with current best practice. • Follow-up arrangements are inadequate.

C. Interpersonal skills	Positive indicators:
• Use of recognised communication techniques that enhance understanding of a patient's illness and promote a shared approach to managing problems. • Practising ethically with respect for equality and diversity in line with accepted codes of professional conduct.	• Displays good listening skills; appears genuinely interested in getting to the heart of the problem. • Develops a *shared* management plan, incorporating the patient's agenda and specific concerns. • Checks understanding and agreement with the patient. Negative indicators: • Interrupts inappropriately, appears judgemental or lacks sympathy. • Uses formulaic questions; the consultation lacks natural flow. • Is doctor-centred; fails to adequately pick up or address verbal or non-verbal cues.

Group debrief

- Assess the doctor's verbal and non-verbal response to the patient presenting with a list. Did the doctor seem genuinely interested in ascertaining the main reason for the patient consulting or did they show their dismay or negative feelings?
- Was there a good mix of open and closed questions to adequately and safely prioritise the focus of the consultation?
- Did the doctor notice and respond to cues at the time they were offered by the patient? Did the doctor repeat back so the patient knew they understood? Did the doctor legitimise the patient's feelings, for example by saying, 'This is clearly worrying you a great deal.'?
- Was there a shared management plan? Did the doctor draw up a list (migraine; impact of headache on work; blood test for thyroid disease) and negotiate which to deal with first?: 'We need to make the best plan we can to sort out these problems. I think we should take each one seriously, giving due time and attention rather than hastily construct a plan.'
- One of the most common feedback statements to CSA failures is 'does not identify the patient's agenda, health beliefs and preferences or does not make use of verbal and non-verbal cues.' In this case, evaluate how well the doctor communicated with a patient presenting with a list of problems. Was the doctor able to provide specific information that moved the consultation forward, having assessed what the patient already knew, what they wanted to know and what they needed to know?

Relevant literature

Gask, L. and Usherwood, T. (2002) ABC of psychological medicine. The consultation. *BMJ*, **324:** 1567. www.bmj.com/content/324/7353/1567

Suchman A.L. *et al.* (1997) A model of empathic communication in the medical interview. *JAMA*, **277(8):** 678–682.

Search www.skillscascade.com/index.html for articles on agenda setting and patient cues.

Practice case 9 – Adult woman

Brief to the patient

- You are Becky Engels, a 28 year old married woman. You are currently 32 weeks pregnant with your first baby. It has been an uneventful pregnancy so far.
- You have come to see the doctor today because you have had a severe 'all over' itch for the last three days. E45 didn't help. If questioned in detail, the itch is worse over your hands and feet, but there is nothing to see.
- You have not been in contact with anything new and you have not come into contact with chickenpox. You don't feel unwell.
- You think the itchiness may be a reaction to the powdered gloves you use at work. You work for a dental laboratory making dentures. Work switched from powdered to non-powdered gloves 4 years ago but you think you are having a delayed reaction to latex.
- You are also having a stressful time at work. Your pregnant work colleague is being allowed to start her maternity leave at 32 weeks because she has symphysis pubis pain. You have been asked to start leave at 38 weeks.
- If offered, you are concerned about using steroid creams and antihistamines while pregnant. You would like a week off work because you are tired and the itch is disrupting your sleep.
- If the doctor offers a blood test or hospital referral, you want to know why. You become concerned that something is wrong. What should you tell your husband? Will you have to start maternity leave soon? What should you tell work?

Patient medical record for the doctor

Name   Rebecca Engels (28 years)

Past medical history   Currently pregnant

Current medication   none

This practice case originally appeared in *GP* and is reproduced here in an amended form with permission (see **www.gponline.com**)

Marking guide for the assessor

Generic indicators for targeted assessment domains	Descriptors – positive and negative
A. Data gathering, technical and assessment skills: • Gathering of data for clinical judgement, choice of examination, investigations and their interpretations. • Demonstrating proficiency in performing physical examinations and using diagnostic and therapeutic instruments.	Positive indicators: • Elicits details of itch, asking if it is worse at night and if it involves palms and soles. Also asks about other evidence of cholestasis such as jaundice, pale stools, dark urine. Possible viral hepatitis and eczema are considered. • Checks that mum is feeling well and baby is kicking (obstetric cholestasis (OC) increases the risk of intrauterine death). • Finds out the patient's ideas about possible latex allergy or sensitivity to powdered gloves and explains why this is unlikely. • Elicits relevant work stressors. • Discovers the patient's expectations for topical treatment and time off work. Negative indicators: • Fails to question sufficiently to explore the possibility of OC. • Assumes this is dry skin or eczema.

B. Clinical management skills	Positive indicators:
• Recognition and management of common medical conditions in primary care. Demonstrates flexible and structured approach to decision-making. • Demonstrating ability to deal with multiple complaints and co-morbidity and to promote a shared approach to managing problems.	• Explains the possibility of OC using jargon-free language, without alarming the patient. • Addresses her concerns about antihistamines and steroid creams. If prescribed, the medication is appropriate and evidence based, with clear instructions on how to use and its safety in pregnancy. • Makes balanced plans: requests the appropriate blood tests (bile salts, LFTs, viral screen) and onward referral for consultant-led care and delivery in a hospital at 37–38 weeks if LFTs and bile acids are abnormal. Negative indicators: • Fails to explain OC. • Fails to discuss the rationale for blood tests / referral or alarms the patient inappropriately. • Prescribes inappropriately.
C. Interpersonal skills	Positive indicators:
• Use of recognised communication techniques that enhance understanding of a patient's illness and promote a shared approach to managing problems. • Practising ethically with respect for equality and diversity in line with accepted codes of professional conduct.	• Displays empathy to her work situation. • Empowers her so she can discuss the issue with her husband and make decisions about her work. • Involves the patient in decisions about blood tests and hospital referral. Negative indicators: • The consultation is doctor-centred: lack of empathy; insufficient information sharing; lack of patient involvement about decisions. • Is underly or overly challenging when negotiating time off work. • Makes judgemental or non-professional statements about her boss, colleagues, or midwife.

Group debrief

- Evaluate whether the doctor gathered sufficient information, from the history and examination, to arrive at a reasonable hypothesis regarding the cause of this patient's itchiness. Were red flags, such as anorexia, jaundice, a bruising tendency and a reduction in foetal movements excluded?
- Did the doctor elicit and address Becky's idea about latex allergy causing her itch; her concerns about the medication or illness harming the baby; and her expectation of a 'sick note'?
- Did the doctor explain the diagnosis and management plan in jargon-free language? Did he refer for specialist advice, discuss that certain blood tests were needed and that birth plans may need revision? Did he provide the information in chunks and check the patient's understanding at each step?
- Evaluate whether the doctor handled the request for a 'sick note' fairly and dealt with the maternity leave issue in a way that encouraged the patient's autonomy.
- Did the doctor involve the patient in decisions and offer the patient options? In some cases, it may be difficult to offer choice, as in this case where a referral to obstetrics is warranted. The doctor could say, 'I think that the safest thing to do is organise blood tests and monitoring of the baby in hospital. How do you feel about that?' This allows the patient to voice any reasons why she cannot go to hospital (such as 'there is nobody at home to look after my step-son when he returns from school'. However, involving the patient in the decision-making provides the opportunity to uncover and deal with potential problems.

Relevant literature

tinyurl.com/CS3e-Pc9a (*takes you to* www.rcog.org.../gtg_43.pdf)

Practice case 10 - Adult man

Brief to the patient

- You are Jake Gibson, a 29 year old married man.
- You have come to see the doctor today because for the last 24 hours, you have been going to the toilet every 1 to 2 hours. You have a 'burning feeling' when you pass urine.
- If questioned in detail, you deny feeling unwell or having a high fever. You do not have diarrhoea or vomiting but you have mild nausea that has prevented you from eating today. You haven't had kidney stones, loin pain or frothy or bloodstained urine.
- If asked, you have not been unfaithful to your wife. Both of you had negative 'VD' screens before commencing your relationship.
- You think you have a bladder infection. When your wife had similar symptoms, she was given a short course of antibiotics.
- You have just been to the toilet while in the waiting room and you definitely cannot produce a urine sample now. You also have an urgent appointment with your bank manager and will find it difficult to return to the surgery later.
- You are a snowboarding instructor for an events company and leave in three days for a 2-week snowboarding job in Austria. You don't know what medical facilities are available at the resort.
- You want some antibiotics, just like your wife was given. You are not allergic to any antibiotics.
- If you are told to bring a sample back, you become impatient because you were told the blood tests and kidney scans done in April last year ruled out any kidney problems.

Patient medical record for the doctor

Name   Jake Gibson (29 years)

Past medical history   Isolated microscopic haematuria (April last year)

Letter from nephrologist (April last year):

'Dear GP
I do not feel that low level microscopic haematuria in the absence of proteinuria, abnormal renal function, hypertension or symptoms requires further investigation. You may consider arranging an ultrasound. I am sure this is likely to be normal but it

is conceivable that you may pick up dysplastic, atrophic or polycystic kidneys. I do not think a renal appointment will add anything.'

Investigations

U&Es (April):	No abnormality
US kidneys (April):	Normal appearances. Both kidneys normal size. No pc dilatation. Normal bladder.

Marking guide for the assessor

Generic indicators for targeted assessment domains	Descriptors – positive and negative
A. Data gathering, technical and assessment skills: • Gathering of data for clinical judgement, choice of examination, investigations and their interpretations. • Demonstrating proficiency in performing physical examinations and using diagnostic and therapeutic instruments.	Positive indicators: • Systematically works through a diagnostic sieve: UTI, STI and kidney stones. • Enquires about Jake's previous investigation for recurrent microscopic haematuria. Understands how Jake's previous negative investigation and his wife's UTI treatment affect his presentation today. • Asks for a urine sample. Note – in the absence of symptoms of systemic illness, marks are not deducted if a more detailed physical examination is omitted. Negative indicators: • Fails to elicit above points. • Assumes this is a UTI; does not take a sexual history.

B. Clinical management skills	Positive indicators:
• Recognition and management of common medical conditions in primary care. Demonstrates flexible and structured approach to decision-making.	• Persuades the patient to drop off an MSU and discusses potential management plans based on either positive or negative results.
• Demonstrating ability to deal with multiple complaints and co-morbidity and to promote a shared approach to managing problems.	• If prescribes, chooses a suitable antibiotic (at correct dose and duration) with clear instructions on how to take the medication. If he tries to negotiate a delayed prescription or no prescription, justifies his reasoning.
	• Provides information about UTIs in men and how their investigation and management differs from UTIs in women.
	Negative indicators:
	• Fails to elicit above points.
	• By failing to adequately explain why an MSU is important, the patient remains unaware or unconvinced of the dangers of not returning with an MSU.
C. Interpersonal skills	Positive indicators:
• Use of recognised communication techniques that enhance understanding of a patient's illness and promote a shared approach to managing problems.	• Shows flexibility and empathy – arranges investigations and treatment around the patient's work commitments.
• Practising ethically with respect for equality and diversity in line with accepted codes of professional conduct.	• Involves the patient in decisions, negotiates an MSU and follow-up.
	• In explaining UTIs in men, uses the patient's ideas about 'bladder infections' and builds on what the patient already knows about the treatment of UTIs in women.
	Negative indicators:
	• Fails to elicit above points.
	• Is didactic – hastily recommends Jake cancel or postpone his trip.
	• Is rigid – lacks sensitivity to the patient's tight timescales.

Group debrief

- Did the doctor elicit and address Jake's idea that there is no difference in the treatment of UTIs in men and women; his concern that further (repetitive) investigations will unnecessarily delay his work trip; and his expectation of immediate antibiotics?
- Did the doctor adequately explain the need for an MSU?
- Evaluate the doctor's response to Jake's reluctance to return later with an MSU. Was he sensitive to Jake's pressured deadlines?
- Evaluate whether the doctor dealt adequately with the uncertainty created by not having an MSU. Was he safe in his management?
- The most common feedback statement to CSA failures is 'does not develop a management plan (including prescription and referral) that is appropriate and in line with current best practice or make arrangements for follow-up and safety netting'. In this case, evaluate whether the doctor formulated a safe management plan for a patient who perceives further investigation as repetitive and time-consuming. The skill in this case is to shift the patient's ideas so that he wants to be investigated further and prioritises getting an MSU to the surgery before leaving on his overseas trip.

Relevant literature

www.sign.ac.uk/pdf/sign88.pdf – pages 16–17.

Practice case 11 – Adult man

Brief to the patient

- You are Robert Williams, a 64 year old engineer.
- You present today, slightly embarrassed but determined, to ask for an erectile dysfunction drug.
- Your wife died two years ago. You started dating a 54-year-old woman three months ago. You have a good relationship but are unable to maintain your erection.
- If asked, you say that you still get erections at night. You have never suffered from premature ejaculation.
- You find your partner attractive, your mood is good, your children like your new partner and you have no financial worries.
- You think that you have 'performance anxiety' and would like to take Viagra. You think that once the cycle is broken, you will not require medication.
- If asked, you are in good health and you have not had previous medical issues or surgery. You are not taking any medication, except for the occasional ibuprofen for back pain. You have no problems with urine flow or frequency. You do not know your family history, having been adopted.
- You have put on 10 kg in the past two years, drink 4 beers three times per week and a bottle of red wine on weekends. You smoke the occasional cigar and do very little exercise.
- If the doctor asks to examine your BP and weight, you hand him a card: 'BP 134/86'; 'weight 90kg; BMI 29'. If an examination of the genitalia is requested, hand over a card: 'normal penis and testes'. Decline a prostate examination.
- You would like a prescription, preferably an NHS script, but you are willing to pay for it. You are worried about the quality of the tablets sold on the internet. You want the script today because you have planned a romantic weekend away.

Patient medical record for the doctor

Name   Robert Williams (64 years)

Past medical history   Mechanical low back pain (2009) – sick note × 1 week
                                Fungal nail infection (2005)

This practice case originally appeared in *GP* and is reproduced here in an amended form with permission (see **www.gponline.com**)

Marking guide for the assessor

Generic indicators for targeted assessment domains	Descriptors – positive and negative
A. Data gathering, technical and assessment skills: • Gathering of data for clinical judgement, choice of examination, investigations and their interpretations. • Demonstrating proficiency in performing physical examinations and using diagnostic and therapeutic instruments.	Positive indicators: • Asks open questions (to explore the medication request and type of sexual problem) followed by closed questions to clarify possible causes of erectile dysfunction (ED) such as cardiovascular problems, depression, endocrine, surgical, medication side effect or psychological issues such as family or financial anxieties. • Enquires about lifestyle: smoking, alcohol, exercise and diet. • Undertakes a targeted examination: BP, weight, penis and testes. In the absence of lower urinary tract symptoms, a prostate examination is deferred. Negative indicators: • Questioning is not sufficiently detailed to exclude organic or psychological causes of ED. • In particular, the opportunity to explore cardiovascular issues and question holistically (including job worries, children, grief) is missed. • The physical examination is not undertaken or is insufficiently targeted.

B. Clinical management skills	Positive indicators:
<ul><li>Recognition and management of common medical conditions in primary care. Demonstrates flexible and structured approach to decision-making.</li><li>Demonstrating ability to deal with multiple complaints and co-morbidity and to promote a shared approach to managing problems.</li></ul>	<ul><li>Discusses further investigation and justifies request for blood tests (fasting glucose, lipids and 9–11 am serum testosterone).</li><li>Management options, including lifestyle changes and drug treatment, are discussed.</li><li>Advises prescription following blood results, but if new medication, such as generic sildenafil, is prescribed, the patient is advised on safe dosing and cautioned about possible side effects.</li><li>Adequate follow-up is arranged.</li></ul> Negative indicators:<ul><li>The investigation of the problem is inadequate or poorly targeted.</li><li>Prescribing behaviour is not in line with NHS policy.</li><li>Generic sildenafil is prescribed on the NHS without explaining the difference between short- and long-acting PDE-5 drugs.</li><li>Patient is inadequately advised about dose, timing, need for sexual stimulation or success rates.</li><li>Follow-up arrangements are inadequate.</li></ul>

C. Interpersonal skills	Positive indicators:
• Use of recognised communication techniques that enhance understanding of a patient's illness and promote a shared approach to managing problems. • Practising ethically with respect for equality and diversity in line with accepted codes of professional conduct.	• Deals with this potentially embarrassing problem sensitively. Questions are asked in a professional manner. • The examination and management is conducted with confidence. • Information about further investigation is delivered concisely, in language that is easily understood. • The patient is provided with opportunities to seek clarification. Negative indicators: • Assumes the patient wants an NHS script and the patient is not given options. • Does not encourage the patient to share his ideas. • Does not negotiate a mutually acceptable plan.

Group debrief

- Some CSA cases are written with the patient asking for something specific. In this case, the patient asks for sildenafil. In other cases, the patient may ask for a referral or a blood test or a procedure, such as a vasectomy. It is important in such cases to explore the patient's reasons for the request.
- It is also imperative to assess if alternative options are more appropriate. In this case, marks are awarded if attention is paid to modifying the patient's lifestyle and assessing his cardiovascular risk as well as negotiating the sildenafil prescription.
- A common reason for failure in the CSA is that the doctor 'does not recognise the challenge (e.g. the patient's problem or ethical dilemma)'.
- Evaluate whether the doctor adequately explored the patient's problem by asking sufficient questions about organic and psycho-social issues.
- Did the doctor ascertain the patient's ideas and address his expectations by discussing the limited success rate of the requested medication? Evaluate whether the ethical dilemma (most PDE-5 drugs are not funded) was negotiated in a supportive and sensitive manner.

Relevant literature

British Society for Sexual Medicine (2007) *Guidelines on the Management of Erectile Dysfunction*: www.bssm.org.uk

Resources for revision

tinyurl.com/CS3e-Pc11a (*takes you to* www.guidelines.co.uk/bssm/erectile-dysfunction)

Practice case 12 – Adult woman

Brief to the patient

- You are Polly Avery, a 28 year old administrative assistant at a local timber merchants, unmarried and single for the last three years.
- You attend today because when you saw the practice nurse for a smear last week, she advised you that it is not good for your health to have only three periods in a year, but she was unable to explain why this is a problem.
- If questioned about how the problem started, you are not sure. You stopped taking the combined pill (Cileste) three years ago. For the first two years, your periods occurred every two months. In the last year, you had a period every four months. Bleeding is light and unpredictable. You are not troubled by the irregular bleeding and until the nurse mentioned it, had not perceived a problem.
- If specifically questioned, you admit to hair growing on your chest and chin, which you remove. You have an oily T-zone but no acne.
- Despite playing rugby, running to keep fit, and attendance at a weekly slimming club, you find it difficult to lose the 12kg you gained three years ago after your relationship ended.
- If asked, you do not have symptoms of diabetes – no excessive thirst or urination or recurrent minor infections.
- You are not in a relationship and fertility is currently not an issue.
- You had ignored these symptoms of scanty, infrequent periods, difficulty losing weight and excessive hairiness on your chin and chest, but the nurse's reaction scared you into asking yourself whether you have a gynaecological problem. Are tests needed? What can you do to improve your health?
- If a family history is taken, you say that your family is healthy, but if polycystic ovarian syndrome (PCOS) is mentioned, you recall that your sister (age 40) may have this. You know very little about PCOS, but you are keen to know more. You would like to read some written information before deciding on a particular treatment.
- If tests are ordered, you want to know what the results could mean. You are concerned that these will affect your insurance. You plan to buy a house soon.
- If weight loss is mentioned, you sigh and appear defeated. It has been a struggle to keep the weight off over the last three years and you are not hopeful about losing more weight.
- If the doctor examines you, the card you hand to him or her states 'BP 134/88, pulse 86, weight 87 kg; BMI 28.'

Patient medical record for the doctor

Name	Polly Avery (28 years)
Past medical history	Thoracic back pain 3 months ago Ankle pain from rugby injury 9 months ago
Past medication	Naproxen 250 mg thrice daily (9 months ago) Omeprazole 20 mg once daily (9 months ago)

Consultation note by Practice Nurse (last week):
'LMP 12 of last month. No previous smear abnormalities. Very irregular menstrual cycle. 4–5 months between periods. Not currently sexually active. Never smoked tobacco.
O/E: medium speculum. Transition zone seen. Smear taken. Nullip – bled slightly on contact. BP 132/80.
Plan: will write to patient with smear results. Advised to see GP to discuss periods.'

Marking guide for the assessor

Generic indicators for targeted assessment domains	Descriptors – positive and negative
A. Data gathering, technical and assessment skills: • Gathering of data for clinical judgement, choice of examination, investigations and their interpretations. • Demonstrating proficiency in performing physical examinations and using diagnostic and therapeutic instruments.	Positive indicators: • Makes use of the medical record provided and gathers sufficient information through the use of open and closed questions to suspect PCOS. • Excludes red flags – asks about other metabolic problems such as diabetes and hypothyroidism. • The doctor is holistic – marital status, plans for a family, and occupation are discussed. • The doctor performs a general examination relevant to supporting or refuting the diagnosis of PCOS. Negative indicators: • Does not systematically gather data from history or examination; makes assumptions about the problem. • Not appropriately selective in choice of examination. • Fails to interpret examination findings correctly.

B. Clinical management skills	Positive indicators:
• Recognition and management of common medical conditions in primary care. Demonstrates flexible and structured approach to decision-making. • Demonstrating ability to deal with multiple complaints and co-morbidity and to promote a shared approach to managing problems.	• The doctor on the basis of probability makes a diagnosis of PCOS. • The explanation of PCOS is in simple, jargon-free language. The doctor checks the patient's understanding periodically. • Management options, including possible blood tests, scans or referral to the practice nurse for nutritional support, are openly discussed. • Management is evidence based and informed by UK guidelines. Negative indicators: • The doctor fails to consider common causes of oligomenorrhoea. • The doctor fails to sufficiently explain what PCOS is to enhance the patient's understanding. • Further investigation and management is not appropriate or inappropriately timed (urgent rather than routine tests are requested). • Follow-up arrangements are inadequate.

C. Interpersonal skills	Positive indicators:
• Use of recognised communication techniques that enhance understanding of a patient's illness and promote a shared approach to managing problems. • Practising ethically with respect for equality and diversity in line with accepted codes of professional conduct.	• Enquires about why the patient presents today – her concerns and expectations are elicited at an early stage. • The doctor shares his or her thoughts and involves the patient in decisions. • By providing explanations that are relevant and understandable, the patient's autonomy and opinions are encouraged. Hence, the management plan, including the possible prescription of hormonal medication, is jointly constructed. • The cue about difficulties with weight is recognised and the doctor responds appropriately. Negative indicators: • The doctor makes assumptions from reading the nurse's notes and fails to inquire about the patient's health understanding or respond to her concerns. • The doctor fails to explore the patient's psychosocial context and assumes that fertility or fears about diabetes drive her presentation today. • The doctor fails to inform or empower the patient to contribute to management decisions; a prescription for hormonal medication or a list for a battery of tests is handed to the patient with inadequate explanation. • The doctor fails to recognise or respond to the cue about weight.

Group debrief

- The most common reason for failure in the CSA is the candidate's failure to develop a management plan.
- This case tests the candidate's ability to recognise and manage the first presentation of oligomenorrhoea. The history taking and examination should be sufficiently selective to arrive at a possible diagnosis of PCOS fairly quickly. It is important to establish which aspect of PCOS will be the priority for treatment. Fertility, hirsutism, diabetes and hypertension are not identified as pressing problems. However, the doctor is aware of the relationship between oligomenorrhoea and endometrial cancer – this aspect of care is prioritised so subsequent discussion about treatment addresses the need to induce withdrawal bleeds every 3–4 months.
- Assess how well the candidate discussed 'PCOS and having very infrequent periods'. Was the explanation jargon-free or did it sound technical or alarming to the patient? Did the doctor discuss possible blood tests or scans? Did the patient understand why these investigations were being requested?
- Did the doctor involve the patient in decisions and offer the patient options? This patient had an expectation of being given information about the condition before deciding on a treatment pathway. Was the doctor able to elicit and respond to this expectation? Or, did the doctor ignore this expectation and try to prescribe in this first consultation a treatment to induce withdrawal bleeds?
- What was the doctor's response to the weight cue? How empathetic was the response? Was the doctor's response 'patient education' or the giving of information, somewhat authoritarian? Or did the doctor try to explore the patient's motivation to lose weight? When the patient revealed her difficulties, was the doctor's response neutral, for example: 'How do you make sense of all of this?' and appropriately reflective: 'Do you see a way to increase your exercise or reduce your calories?'? The high-scoring candidate in the 'Interpersonal Skills' section demonstrates good motivational interviewing skills: an open style that allows the patient to explore her strategies for overcoming barriers to change; agenda setting; open questions; reflective listening and affirmations.

Relevant literature

For an excellent overview of the management of PCOS, see:
Harding E (2010) Polycystic Ovarian Syndrome, *InnovAiT*, **3 (2):** 71–75.
doi: 10.1093/innovait/inp124

To develop your motivational interviewing skills, see:
Storr E (2011) Motivational interviewing: a positive approach, *InnovAiT,* **4(9):** 533–538.
doi:10.1093/innovait/inr045

Practice case 13 – Adult man

Brief to the patient

- You are Martin Stander, a 28 year old unmarried man who works as a coordinator for a local logistics company. You attend to ask the doctor for a referral to the practice counsellor for 'help with my drinking'.
- Your drinking has increased over the last six weeks and you have got into trouble twice with the police. On these two occasions, you got into fights and on the last occasion you had to be restrained, hence the bruises on your face today. The police hearings are set for a week and a month away. The police have told you that you are 'throwing your life and career away'. You want to take their advice and seek help with your drinking.
- The fights were unprovoked. Nobody was seriously injured because you 'lose all coordination when drunk'.
- If specifically asked whom you are angry with, you say 'with life and circumstances'. Your girlfriend is 4 months pregnant with your child. You feel uncertain about getting married and think you are too young to become a father. You feel angry about the contraception failure.
- Your girlfriend plans to move in with you into your parents' house because you cannot afford to live on your own. Your parents have been supportive. Although you haven't decided to marry as yet, you feel your mum will become attached to the baby and it will be difficult to part ways after the baby's birth. Your girlfriend, after the last fight, asked if you wanted her to move out. You are working things through. You have been in a steady relationship for 11 months. Your girlfriend attends the local teacher training college. Her family live two hours' drive away.
- Your older brother married young (age 19) and divorced three years later. He has experienced difficulty in seeing his children. Your mother often says she feels sad that her grandchildren 'are strangers to her'.
- You are a good rugby player and your social life revolves around the local rugby club. You usually binge after rugby matches, but restrict your intake to less than 20 units per week. Over the last 6 weeks, you drank 'way more than this' and try to pass out so you don't have to think about your situation.
- Your main symptom is anxiety about your future. You do not have symptoms of depression – no sleep disturbance, loss of appetite or weight, feelings of guilt or poor self-esteem or apathy or excessive tiredness.
- You would like to speak to someone 'to sort out my head' and you expect a referral to the practice counsellor.
- If the doctor discusses Alcoholics Anonymous with you, you say that you are not an alcoholic and don't think their service is appropriate to your needs.

- If signposted to local services (Relate or social services), you want to know how these services could be useful to you.
- If the doctor arranges a follow-up appointment, you want to know when and why you should attend. With the court appearances, you do not want to take too much time off work.

Patient medical record for the doctor

Name   Martin Stander (28 years)

Social and family history   Unmarried
                                Works for a logistics company
                                Plays 1st row for the local amateur rugby club

Past medical history   Hayfever (every spring)
                                Left AC joint injury (5 months ago)
                                Right ACL reconstruction (2 years ago)

Past medication   Loratidine 10 mg daily (spring)

Marking guide for the assessor

Generic indicators for targeted assessment domains	Descriptors – positive and negative
A. Data gathering, technical and assessment skills: • Gathering of data for clinical judgement, choice of examination, investigations and their interpretations. • Demonstrating proficiency in performing physical examinations and using diagnostic and therapeutic instruments.	Positive indicators: • Asks selective questions, tailored to establishing whether hazardous drinking has occurred (e.g. FAST screening). Takes a comprehensive alcohol and drug history. • Checks if there are reasons (legal, occupational, insurance) why the patient may under-report alcohol consumption. Sufficient information is gathered to decide if adjunctive biological tests are needed. • Enquires about red flags, such as deliberate self-harm (DSH) and risk to others (domestic violence) from the patient's drinking. • Picks up the physical cue (facial bruise) – gathers information about recent fights / police involvement that leads to a deeper understanding of the patient's presentation today. • Details of the patient's support network are obtained. Negative indicators: • Questioning is not sufficiently selective. By the end of the history taking, the doctor is unable to quantify the extent of the drinking problem. • By the end of the history taking, the doctor is unable to decide whether adjunctive biological tests (GGT, MCV) are needed. • Assessment is not holistic – important information about work, hobbies (rugby) or family life (pregnant girlfriend moving in with mother who yearns for close relationship with grandchild) is missed.

B. Clinical management skills	Positive indicators:
• Recognition and management of common medical conditions in primary care. Demonstrates flexible and structured approach to decision-making. • Demonstrating ability to deal with multiple complaints and co-morbidity and to promote a shared approach to managing problems.	• The doctor makes a diagnosis – harmful drinking and using the patient's ideas and beliefs, feeds this back to the patient. • Management options, including abstinence or cutting down with goals of reduction, are jointly agreed. • While support networks and external agencies are discussed, the patient's personal responsibility for change is emphasised. • Review is planned: to offer encouragement, monitoring (MVC/GGT) or reassess (the costs and benefits of change). Negative indicators: • Doctors fail to manage safely or in line with current best practice. • Follow-up arrangements are inadequate.
C. Interpersonal skills	Positive indicators:
• Use of recognised communication techniques that enhance understanding of a patient's illness and promote a shared approach to managing problems. • Practising ethically with respect for equality and diversity in line with accepted codes of professional conduct.	• The doctor displays the skill of empathic interviewing: listening reflectively without cajoling or confronting; exploring with the patient the reasons for change as he sees his situation. • The doctor makes reflective statements and summarises periodically to check and convey understanding. • Personal responsibility is emphasised but the doctor supports the patient. • Statements are neutral and non-judgemental, thereby enhancing the patient's belief in their ability to change. Negative indicators: • The doctor does not listen attentively – seems distracted, pre-occupied or focused on uncovering a different (hidden) agenda. • The doctor gives advice, lectures or educates, potentially creating a parent–child dynamic. • The doctor appears judgemental or unhopeful about the patient's ability to change.

Group debrief

In this case, the doctor's main task is to empower the patient to self-care. On the surface, this appears to be a simple case – harmful alcohol usage. The patient's request for a referral to the practice counsellor is not unreasonable. The challenge in this case is the interpersonal skill – how good is the doctor at demonstrating skills to transform holistic understanding of the presenting problem into practical measures to move the patient forward? The motivational interviewing skills touched on in the previous case (PCOS) are also tested here.

With regard to interpersonal skills, assess whether the doctor:
- Asked questions to uncover relevant information outside the patient's current awareness: 'What might be the pros and cons of abstinence?'
- Accurate listening and empathic reflections: 'You sound confused about your girlfriend moving in with your parents.'
- Summarising/recapping information: 'to summarise what we have talked about so far...'
- Synthesising questions that ask the patient to apply the new information discovered to their original belief/behaviour: 'So on the one hand we talked about abstinence and on the other hand we spoke about cutting down. What do you make of it so far?'

Assess if the doctor, by the style of his or her consulting, strengthened the patient's desire to reduce drinking? Did the doctor make statements such as:
- What would you advise someone in your position to do?
- What would you do differently the next time you feel frustrated?
- How might we ensure this happens?
- How shall we handle any setbacks?

Relevant literature

For a brief overview on the philosophy of Motivational Interviewing and the stages of change, see:
www.youtube.com/watch?v=4uUAELqp_9s. You can skip the first two minutes!

For an example of a five minute interview, see:
www.youtube.com/watch?v=dm-rJJPCuTE.

tinyurl.com/CS3e-Pc13a (*takes you to* www.bmj.com/bmj/section-pdf/186224?path=/bmj/342/7795/Practice.full.pdf)

Practice case 14 – Adult woman

Brief to the patient

- You are Kelly Carroll, a 45 year old woman. You present today, two weeks after having had some blood tests, to discuss the results. You definitely fasted for the blood test.
- The doctor who requested the blood tests was checking hormone levels to see if you are menopausal. He also thought that while blood was being taken, you should have some 'general MOT tests'.
- If asked, your mood swings and tiredness started 6 months ago. Little things, like someone leaving the toothpaste uncapped, upset you to the point of tears. You know that your reaction to minor issues is disproportional but you cannot seem to control your anger, irritation and hurt.
- You thought you were not coping with the added responsibility of studying nursing as a mature student so you discontinued the studies and took up a nursing assistant post at the hospice instead.
- You think your symptoms are due to 'stress'. Several issues cause 'stress': feeling lonely at home now that your second teenage daughter has left home to start university; doing menial, boring, repetitive housework; and dealing with dying people at work.
- Your husband, who is nine years younger than you, is busy working towards a promotion. You have spoken to him but feel that he has 'not listened'.
- If asked, you have not had regular periods; only occasional light bleeds since your endometrial ablation six months ago. This makes you feel even less of a woman. You also have hot flushes perhaps once or twice per week but you feel you can cope with them. However, you are tired, despite 8 hours of sleep, and would like to have more energy.
- If the doctor discusses HRT with you, you would like to know the pros and cons of HRT. You do not have contra-indications to HRT, but wonder if you are at increased risk of breast cancer as your mum's sister had breast cancer at age 52.
- If anti-depressants are discussed, you want to know if the doctor thinks 'it is all in my head'.
- You have come across alternative medications at the hospice and you are keen on 'natural remedies'. You would like more information on natural treatments for the menopause. You have read that phyto-oestrogens can be helpful but want the doctor's opinion.

Patient medical record for the doctor

Name   Kelly Carroll (45 years)

Past medical history   Endometrial ablation (6 months ago)
                                  Menorrhagia (2 years ago)
                                  Post-natal depression (9 years ago)

Past medication   zoladex implant 3.6 mg (6 months ago)

Consultation note by Dr Brown (4 weeks ago):
'Menopausal symptoms: hot flushes, feeling irritable, vaginal dryness, reduced energy and reduced sleep, waking early and ruminating. Has a stressful job at hospice. Finding it difficult not having periods after ablation. O/E: anxious lady with some pressure of speech. Near to tears at one point. Plan: for FSH, LH, progestogen and cholesterol bloods. ?menopause ?low mood worsening symptoms.'

Blood tests	Tests were done two weeks ago
Fasting glucose	6.2 (3–5.5)
Total cholesterol	6.5 mmol/l
HDL	1.2
Plasma oestradiol	42 pmol/l (40–1930)
Serum progestogen	1 mmol/l (14–90)
Plasma prolactin	77 mIU/l (60–620)
Plasma FSH	42 IU/l (1.5–33)
Plasma LH	32.5 IU/l (2–10)
TSH (2 years ago)	3.64 mIU/l (0.35–5.5)

Marking guide for the assessor

Generic indicators for targeted assessment domains	Descriptors – positive and negative
A. Data gathering, technical and assessment skills: • Gathering of data for clinical judgement, choice of examination, investigations and their interpretations. • Demonstrating proficiency in performing physical examinations and using diagnostic and therapeutic instruments.	Positive indicators: • Asks selective questions, tailored to establishing whether on balance, mood symptoms are most likely due to the menopause or to depression. • Enquires about red flags, such as deliberate self harm (DSH). Also takes an alcohol and drug history. • How the patient feels about the diagnosis and her commitment to different treatment options is explored in some depth. • Enquires about the raised isolated fasting blood glucose and explores possible causes. Negative indicators: • Questioning and mental state examination is not sufficiently selective. If red flags were present, the doctor would be more focused on safely treating depression. By excluding 'red flags', the doctor is able to offer a menu of treatment options. • The doctor fails to explore the patient's 'buy-in' to the diagnosis and consequently the issues arising from her preference for one treatment over an alternative is inadequately considered. • Details of the patient's family life and occupation are not obtained; the assessment is not holistic.

B. Clinical management skills	Positive indicators:
• Recognition and management of common medical conditions in primary care. Demonstrates flexible and structured approach to decision-making. • Demonstrating ability to deal with multiple complaints and co-morbidity and to promote a shared approach to managing problems.	• Doctors discuss what they feel are reasonable treatment options (ride it out, SSRIs, HRT, natural remedies) and explain their reasoning. • The pros and cons of the various management options are discussed. Information on HRT and breast cancer risk is explained in language the patient understands. • The patient is actively involved in the management plan and having obtained sufficient information from the doctor, makes an informed decision on treatment and follow-up. • Doctors arrange for appropriate investigation of the raised fasting glucose. Negative indicators: • Doctors fail to discuss treatment options in a manner that enables the patient to make informed decisions. Doctors may use jargon or technical language. • The patient is not managed safely or in line with current best practice. Some of the treatment options offered are unorthodox or unconventional to UK practice. • Follow-up arrangements are inadequate.

| C. Interpersonal skills
• Use of recognised communication techniques that enhance understanding of a patient's illness and promote a shared approach to managing problems.
• Practising ethically with respect for equality and diversity in line with accepted codes of professional conduct. | Positive indicators:
• The doctor displays empathy and understanding of how the patient's symptoms affect her relationships, work and self-perception.
• The doctor communicates effectively – he or she addresses the specific concerns about HRT and breast cancer and the patient's reluctance to be viewed as a 'head case'.
• The doctor fulfils the patient's expectation for advice about 'natural' menopausal remedies.
• The doctor and patient develop a shared management plan – the patient buys in to the diagnosis and management.

Negative indicators:
• The doctor fails to explore the patient's reluctance to accept a diagnosis of 'menopause'.
• By failing to appreciate her desire to see this as a 'stress problem' to be treated by changing to a phyto-oestrogen rich diet, the doctor may be accused of 'medicalising' the issue and treating with 'pills'. The doctor behaves in a paternalistic manner.
• The doctor appears judgemental or dismissive about the use of natural remedies, which seems at odds with the medical philosophy of the hospice at which she works. |

Group debrief

Was the doctor able to complete his or her essential tasks? Did he or she safely and adequately manage the mood symptoms with sufficient patient involvement and did the doctor act on the isolated raised fasting glucose?

Discuss how the doctor could, if needed, improve his or her performance. In particular, assess whether the doctor:
- established rapport? If so, how?
- addressed Mrs Carroll's specific concerns about breast cancer and being perceived as a 'head case'? If so, how?
- addressed Mrs Carroll's expectations for information on natural remedies for the menopause?
- discussed the evidence base for HRT and natural remedies using simple and jargon-free language?
- involved the patient in the management plan?

Doctors with good interpersonal skills actively elicit the patient's ideas ('I am stressed. I don't think I'm menopausal – that means I'm old'; her concerns (If HRT will help me, how safe is it?') and expectations ('Could natural remedies be equally helpful?'). They incorporate the patient's beliefs into their management plan. If this patient did not buy in to the diagnosis of menopause, how likely is she to comply with a prescription for HRT or SSRIs? What is the harm associated in trying natural remedies for a short period of time? If the patient was not actively involved in the management plan, suggest how the consultation could be made more patient centred.

Relevant literature

http://www.emedicine.com/med/topic3756.htm

Diagnosis and management of menopause: summary of NICE guidance. *BMJ* (2015) **351:** h5746.
tinyurl.com/CS3e-Pc14a (*takes you to* www.bmj.com/...)

Practice case 15 – Adult woman

Brief to the patient

- You are Kay Northrop, a 35 year old married bookkeeper. You attend today because you have had right and middle lower abdominal pain for three days. Although the pain is intermittent, the spasms develop and reach a peak (8/10) before subsiding to a dull ache. This pattern has occurred every few hours for the last three days and seems to be getting worse, rather than better. It does not feel like your IBS pain. You do not feel pregnant.
- The only other symptom is vaginal bleeding, which started 20 days ago. Initially you assumed this was your period, but the bleeding, though light, has continued, mainly in the form of spotting, requiring the use of a panty-liner. Your usual cycle is 4 to 6 days of bleeding every 30 days. You assumed you were bleeding for longer than usual because you missed two periods.
- You do not have urinary frequency, dysuria, diarrhoea or vomiting. You were able to eat today; no nausea or upset tummy.
- You think 'something is wrong' and suspect appendicitis or a miscarriage. You are worried about having a miscarriage. Your husband is in a meeting in Belfast. You are worried about calling him and disrupting his meeting if you have a minor ailment. On the other hand, you are scared about having a miscarriage or being admitted into hospital without him.
- You expect to be told what is wrong with you, how serious it is and how it should be treated. You need sufficient information to decide whether you should ask your husband to shorten his business trip and return home tonight.
- When you saw Dr Brown 3 weeks ago, you were advised to have a blood test 7 days before your next period was due but you started bleeding two days later, so the test was not done.
- If the doctor asks to test your urine, you produce a piece of paper: 'Urine pregnancy test positive. Dipstix: trace leucocytes but no nitrites or protein.'
- If the doctor offers to perform a pelvic examination, you decline (you don't want to be examined while bleeding) unless absolutely necessary. If the doctor convinces you that by examining you, he or she will be able to make a diagnosis, you permit the examination and produce a card: 'Os closed. Tender in right adnexa but no mass palpated. No peritonism.'
- If the doctor checks your pulse and BP, you produce a card: 'pulse 84 regular; BP 132/88.'

Patient medical record for the doctor

Name   Kay Northrop (35 years)

Social and family history   Married 2 years ago. No children

Past medical history   Pre-pregnancy counselling (3 weeks ago)
                                   Irritable bowel syndrome (3 months ago)

Past medication   Mebeverine 135 mg thrice daily × 100T (3 months ago)

Consultation note by Dr Brown (3 weeks ago):
'Stopped Microgynon 12 months ago. Actively trying for a baby for past 8 months. LMP: three months ago. Missed last two periods and then has a bleed lasting 24 hours. After the second missed period, two pregnancy tests were negative. Recent blood tests, including hormone profile, were fine. No past history of STIs or pelvic infection or surgery. Plan: get 21 day progestogen. In view of age (and husband is 38; neither have had children) refer to fertility clinic at next appointment.'

Marking guide for the assessor

Generic indicators for targeted assessment domains	Descriptors – positive and negative
A. Data gathering, technical and assessment skills: • Gathering of data for clinical judgement, choice of examination, investigations and their interpretations. • Demonstrating proficiency in performing physical examinations and using diagnostic and therapeutic instruments.	Positive indicators: • Asks open questions (to explore the nature of the pelvic pain and bleeding) followed by closed questions to clarify LMP and sequence of events. • Asks about red flags: obtains information to assess if this could be a miscarriage, ectopic pregnancy or appendicitis. • If hypovolaemic shock were found on examination, it would add weight to an emergency presentation of ectopic pregnancy. The normal pulse and BP are reassuring. • The most important examination is the pregnancy test. There are arguments for and against performing a vaginal examination (VE). Consider whether performing a VE in a suspected miscarriage or ectopic pregnancy contributes much to the clinical picture. Negative indicators: • Does not systematically gather data from history or examination; makes assumptions about the problem. • Not appropriately selective in choice of examination. • Fails to interpret examination findings correctly.

B. Clinical management skills	Positive indicators:
• Recognition and management of common medical conditions in primary care. Demonstrates flexible and structured approach to decision-making. • Demonstrating ability to deal with multiple complaints and co-morbidity and to promote a shared approach to managing problems.	• The doctor explains the most likely causes of vaginal bleeding with pain in early pregnancy (bleeding in early normal pregnancy / miscarriage / ectopic) in jargon-free language. • Management options, including same or next day appointment in Early Pregnancy Unit (EPU), with early blood tests or scanning, are openly discussed. • Management, including what to do if the pain or bleeding worsens, is discussed. The patient is given sufficient information about best and worst case scenarios to decide on whether or not she interrupts her husband's business trip. Negative indicators: • Doctors fail to consider common conditions in the differential diagnosis or fail to explain these conditions sufficiently to enhance the patient's understanding. • Further investigation and management is not selective. • Decisions about referral are inappropriate or ill timed. • Safety-netting or follow-up arrangements are inadequate.

C. Interpersonal skills • Use of recognised communication techniques that enhance understanding of a patient's illness and promote a shared approach to managing problems. • Practising ethically with respect for equality and diversity in line with accepted codes of professional conduct.	Positive indicators: • The doctor explores the patient's agenda; he or she identifies the patient's ideas about miscarriage or appendicitis; her concerns about being alone in hospital and her expectations for sufficient information to recall her husband if needed. • The doctor explores the patient's ambivalence to VE; is empathetic, non-judgemental and respectful when discussing this with her. He or she provides an explanation of why the examination is chosen/not chosen. • The doctor discusses what he or she feels is the safest action (same or next day appointment in the EPU). However, if the patient expresses a strong preference for being assessed at a later date, when her husband is present, he or she negotiates with the patient to construct a shared management plan, which includes good safety-netting. Negative indicators: • Doctors fail to share their thoughts about the possible diagnosis and the need to manage risk well. The patient is not provided with sufficient information to be meaningfully involved in making decisions. • The doctor seems frustrated or irritated by the patient's reluctance to have a VE and responds negatively. • The doctor instructs the patient; the patient's wishes are not explored or considered in the management decisions.

Group debrief

The most common reason for failure in the CSA is the candidate's failure to develop a management plan. This case tests the candidate's ability to recognise and manage a case of pelvic pain and vaginal bleeding. The differential diagnosis includes bleeding in an early normal pregnancy; however, it is difficult to exclude a miscarriage or an ectopic pregnancy on clinical grounds. Also, the patient's social support is minimal. The doctor needs to suspect an ectopic pregnancy (red flag), broach the possibility of bad news, support her and deal with the emergency.

Discuss how the doctor could, if needed, improve his or her performance. In particular, assess whether the doctor:

- identified the patient's problem with an appropriate opening question, e.g. 'What can I do for you today?'
- established dates and sequence of events
- encouraged the patient to express her feelings?
- demonstrated appropriate confidence?
- assessed the patient's prior knowledge before giving information and gave explanations after discovering the extent of patient's wish for information?
- checked with the patient whether plans were accepted and if concerns were addressed?
- explained seriousness, expected outcome, short- and long-term consequences?
- safety-netted by explaining possible unexpected outcomes and clarified when and how to seek help?

This case specifically tests the doctor's ability to develop a safe, evidence-based management plan. Bearing this in mind, assess whether the doctor was able to establish a differential diagnosis, recognise the need for further investigation and arrange for appropriate help within the allocated time?

Relevant literature

For an overview of the management of bleeding in early pregnancy, see:
Rawal N *et al.* (2009) Bleeding in early pregnancy. *InnovAiT*, **2 (5):** 277–283. doi:10.1093/innovait/inp053

RCOG (2016) Diagnosis and management of ectopic pregnancy. Green-top guideline no. 21 – tinyurl.com/CS3e-Pc15a (*takes you to* www.rcog.org.uk/.../gtg21/)